The Tourniquet Manual
– Principles and Practice

Springer
London
Berlin
Heidelberg
New York
Hong Kong
Milan
Paris
Tokyo

Leslie Klenerman

The Tourniquet Manual – Principles and Practice

Springer

Leslie Klenerman, MBBCh, ChM, FRCSEd, FRCSEng
Emeritus Professor of Orthopaedic and Accident Surgery, University of Liverpool, Liverpool, UK

British Library Cataloguing in Publication Data
Klenerman, Leslie
    The tourniquet manual : principles and practice
    1. Tourniquets
    I. Title
    617.9′178
    ISBN 1852337060

Library of Congress Cataloging-in-Publication Data
Klenerman, Leslie.
    The tourniquet manual : principles and practice/Leslie Klenerman.
        p. ; cm.
    Includes bibliographical references and index.
    ISBN 1-85233-706-0 (alk. paper)
    1. Tourniquets–Handbooks, manuals, etc. I. Title.
    [DNLM: 1. Hemostatic Techniques. 2. Tourniquets. 3. Extremities–surgery.
    4. Intraoperative Complications–prevention & control. 5. Orthopedic Procedures–methods.
    6. Postoperative Complications–prevention & control. 7. Tourniquets–adverse effects.
WH 310 K644t 2003]
RD73.T6K54 2003
617′.9–dc21   2003045601

ISBN 1-85233-706-0 Springer-Verlag London Berlin Heidelberg
a member of BertelsmannSpringer Science+Business Media GmbH
http://www.springer.co.uk

Typeset by Florence Production, Stoodleigh, Devon, England
Printed in the United States of America
28/3830-543210 Printed on acid-free paper SPIN 10896266

Acknowledgements

This book could not have been started without the generous sponsorship of the Medical Defence Union, the Medical Protection Society, the British Association for Surgery of the Knee, the British Orthopaedic Foot Surgery Society, and Anetic Aid, a manufacturer of tourniquets. I am very grateful to these bodies for their help in making this book possible.

Thanks are also due to my wife Naomi and my son Paul for their constant help, criticism and encouragement; to Professor Malcolm Jackson of the Department of Medicine, University of Liverpool, for help with biochemistry; to Derek Eastwood, John Kirkup and Durai Nayagam for their useful comments and corrections; to Alun Jones and Andrew Biggs in the Photographic Department at the Robert Jones and Agnes Hunt Hospital, Oswestry, for invaluable help with the illustrations; and to Stephen White for allowing me access to the theatre during his operation list.

Contents

Introduction

Why write a book on the tourniquet? The tourniquet is used routinely in operating theatres throughout the world, but as far as I know there is no single book that surveys the considerable literature that has accumulated. If used sensibly, the tourniquet is a safe instrument. Most of the few complications seen with its use are preventable. However, when something untoward happens, the tourniquet suddenly becomes an interesting subject, particularly if there is the likelihood of medicolegal consequences. This book summarises the scientific background of the tourniquet and describes a safe physiological approach to preventing complications. Examples of medicolegal problems are included.

Considerable progress had been made since Lister first excised a tuberculous wrist joint in a bloodless field. Many researchers have studied the effects of ischaemia and pressure on nerves and muscles. Tourniquets have entered the age of computers and are now much more sophisticated. Despite this, there is still much dogma surrounding the tourniquet in operating theatres and in textbooks. This book is aimed at orthopaedic surgeons, anaesthetists and operating-theatre staff.

I hope that this short text will stimulate a more widespread interest in the tourniquet and improve safe practice.

Leslie Klenerman
June 2003

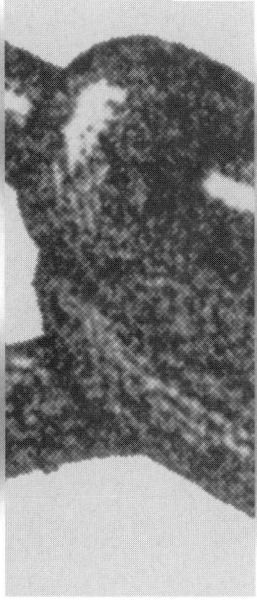

Chapter 1
Historical Background

THE EARLY DEVELOPMENT of the tourniquet is bound up with the operation of amputation. It was only about 140 years ago that the tourniquet was first used in other operations on the limbs. The introduction of the bloodless field was a landmark in the development of orthopaedic operative technique, and it is interesting to recall how this came about.

There is evidence that limbs were amputated as far back as the Neolithic age. Hippocrates recommended cutting through the dead limb at a joint, "care being taken not to wound any living part".[1] Only since Roman times have various constricting devices been employed to help the control of haemorrhage during amputation. Archigenes and Heliodorus, who practised in Rome in the early part of the second century AD, used narrow bands of cloth placed directly above and below the line of incision, each passed two or three times about the limb and tied in a single knot. This mainly controlled the venous bleeding. Heliodorus then relied on tight bandaging of the stump.

For the next 1500 years, no significant alteration appears to have been made in this practice. Ambroise Paré in the sixteenth century advocated tying "a strong or broad fillet like that which women usually bind up their haire withall" above the site of amputation.[2] This helped to retain the maximum length of skin and muscle for the stump, controlled haemorrhage, and reduced pain. The use of a stick to twist the constricting bandage was known to William Fabry of Hilden (1560–1624), although Morell in the Siege of Besançon (1674) is often given credit for this (Figure 1.1). In a work entitled *Currus Triumphalis e Terebintho*, James Yonge of Plymouth gave an account of a similar instrument he had produced.[3] Although Morell's tourniquet was crude, it provided the basis for the greatly improved instrument devised by another Frenchman, Jean Louis Petit (1674–1750; Figure 1.2), in the early part of the next

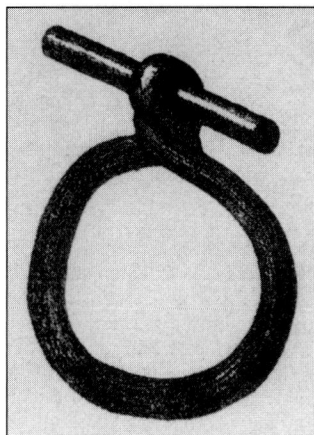

Figure 1.1 Morell-type tourniquet. Reproduced by permission of the Wellcome Library, London, from Seerig, AWH (1838). *Armamentarium Chirurgicium*. Wrocław: A. Gosohorsky.

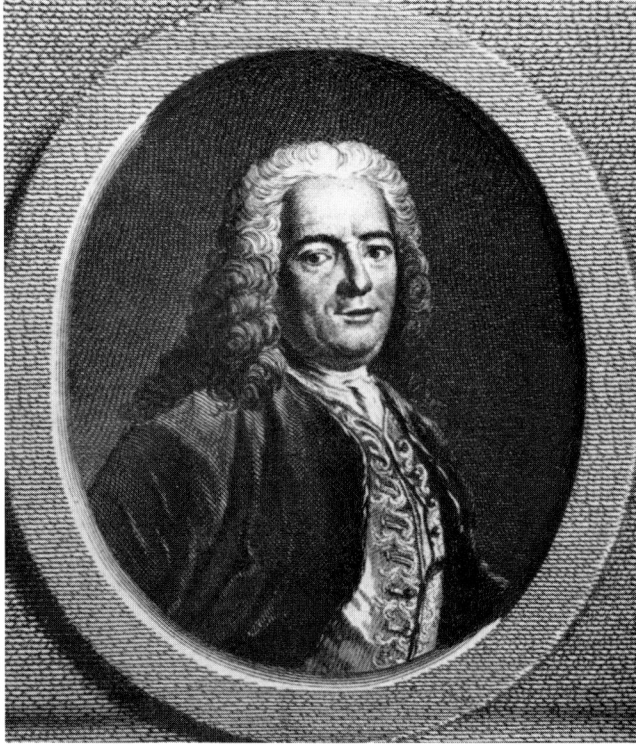

Figure 1.2 Jean Louis Petit. Reproduced by kind permission of the President and Council of the Royal College of Surgeons of England.

century. There were various modifications: according to Chelius, "a pad stuffed with hair, a strong bandage, an ell and a half or two ells long, a stick of tough wood, and a piece of leather, which has on both sides a cut for the passage of the bandage", allowed more precise pressure on the main artery of the limb.[4]

1.1 Screw Tourniquet

Jean Louis Petit, the foremost surgeon in Paris during the first half of the eighteenth century, described his invention of the screw tourniquet before the Academie Royal des Sciences in Paris in 1718. He was the first to use the term "tourniquet", which is derived from the French *tourner* (to turn).[5] His tourniquet was a definite advance because it did not require an assistant to hold the instrument in place, and it could be released readily and reapplied instantly. The tourniquet consisted of a strap that passed around the limb and to which the screw portion was attached. When the screw was tightened, pressure was brought to bear over the main vessel of the limb by a curved piece fixed to the screw. The first screws were made of wood, but later they were made of brass (Figures 1.3 and 1.4). Various modifications of Petit's apparatus remained in use until the latter part of the nineteenth century. However,

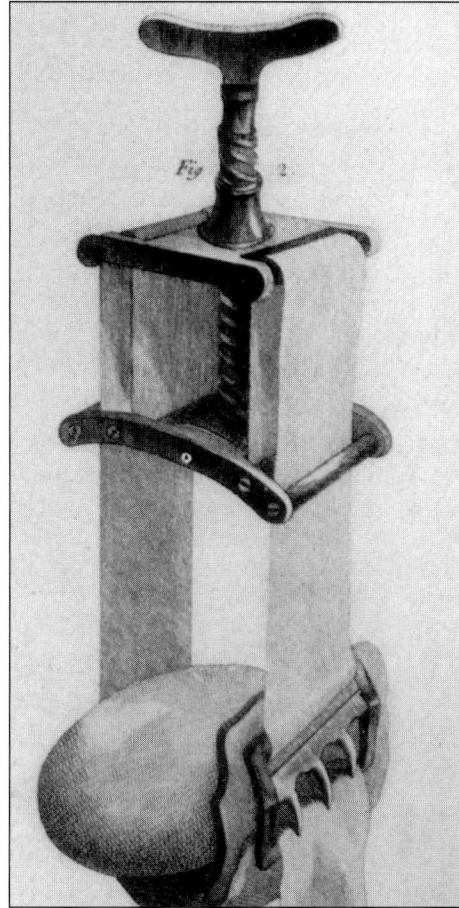

Figure 1.3 Petit's tourniquet. Reproduced with permission of the Wellcome Library, London, from Savigny, JH (1798). *A Collection of Engravings. The Most Modern and Approved Instruments Used in the Practice of Surgery.* The Letter Press by T. Bensley.

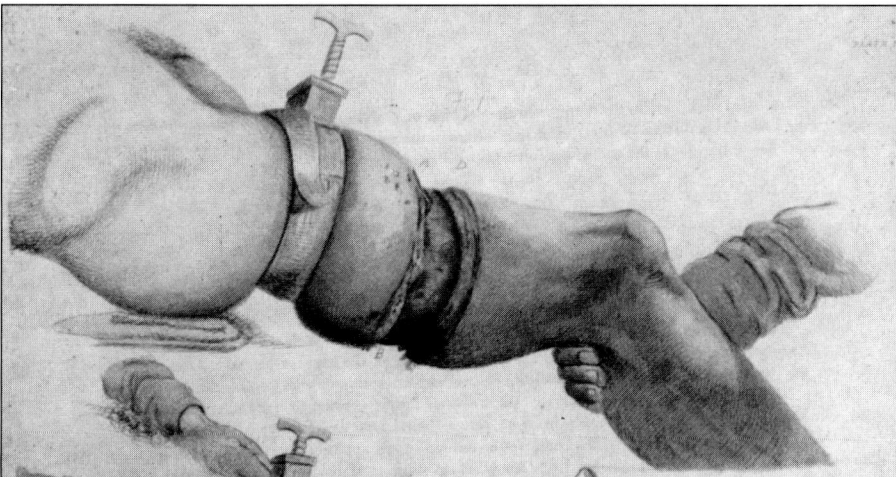

Figure 1.4 Screw tourniquet in place. Reproduced by kind permission of the President and Council of the Royal College of Surgeons of England from Sir Charles Bell (1821). *Illustrations of the Great Operations of Surgery.* London: Longman, Hurst, Rees, Orme and Brown.

during the Crimean War, the British army reverted to using the simpler strap-and-buckle tourniquet.[5]

1.2 Listerian Methods

Joseph Lister (Figure 1.5), in the 1860s, was the first surgeon to use the bloodless field for operations other than amputation, "long before the rest of the world had grasped the idea of operating bloodlessly".[6] He described how his attention had first been directed to this subject when trying to work out a satisfactory method for excision of the wrist joint in tuberculosis to save the hand from amputation and to overcome the profuse bleeding associated with the procedure[7]:

> And I found that when the hand was raised to the utmost degree and kept so for a
> few minutes and then while the elevated position was still maintained, a common
> tourniquet was applied to the arm being screwed up as rapidly as possible, so as to

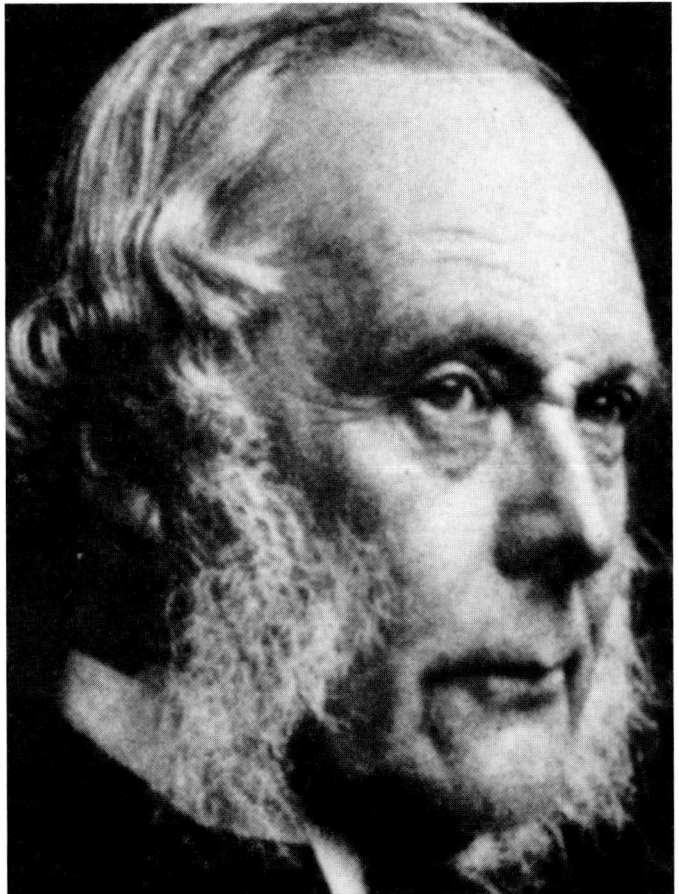

Figure 1.5 Lord Lister

arrest all circulation in the limb and at the same time avoid venous turgescence, I had practically a bloodless field to operate on and thus gained the double advantage of avoiding haemorrhage and inspecting precisely the part with which I was dealing.

Lister emphasised the importance of elevation of the limb before the tourniquet was applied. He considered four minutes to be the best time to empty the blood from the limb. There was thus drainage of all the venous blood and, in addition, arteriolar constriction. Lister gave experimental evidence to prove this point, based on observations on his own hand and on the exposed metacarpal artery of a horse.[7]

1.3 Esmarch's Bandage

Credit for the method of winding a strip of tensile material around the limb is usually given to Johann T. Friederich August von Esmarch (1823–1908; Figure 1.6), Professor of Surgery at Kiel. Von Esmarch was not the first person to use such a device: he gave credit to Sartorius (in 1806), Brunninghausen (in 1818) and Sir Charles Bell (in 1821) for having used methods of expressing venous blood from a limb in combination with a tourniquet.[8] Von Esmarch also acknowledged that Grandesso-Sylvestri in 1871 had used an elastic bandage to empty a limb of blood before amputation. The original Esmarch bandage was a rubber tube the thickness of a finger, wound tightly around the limb to serve as a tourniquet after the blood had been expressed from it by bandaging (Figure 1.7). The "Esmarch bandage" used today was actually designed by von Langenbeck, based on equipment used by Esmarch; correctly, it is termed a "Langenbeck bandage".[9] Esmarch had been bandaging limbs firmly before amputation since 1855, in an effort to conserve blood because he had been disturbed at the amount of blood still present in an amputated limb after it had been severed from the patient. Subsequently, he adopted the technique for other operations on the limb.

In *The Surgeon's Handbook on the Treatment of Wounded in War*, Esmarch gives full details of his technique[10]:

> Operations on the extremities can be performed without loss of blood if they have previously been made bloodless in the following manner:
>
> 1 After the wounds or ulcers, which be present, have been well covered with some waterproof material (varnished paper) the limb is firmly bandaged with an elastic roller from the tips of the fingers or toes upwards till it has reached beyond the site of operation: by this means the blood is completely driven out of the vessels.
>
> 2 Where the bandage ends, an India rubber tube (elastic ligature) is wound with moderately strong traction several times around the limb, so that no more blood can pass through the arteries. The ends of he tube are fastened together by a knot or a hook and chain.
>
> 3 The arteries can be compressed in most cases by an elastic bandage, firmly applied in many circular turns and at the end fastened with a safety pin (van Langenbeck's Schnurbinde).

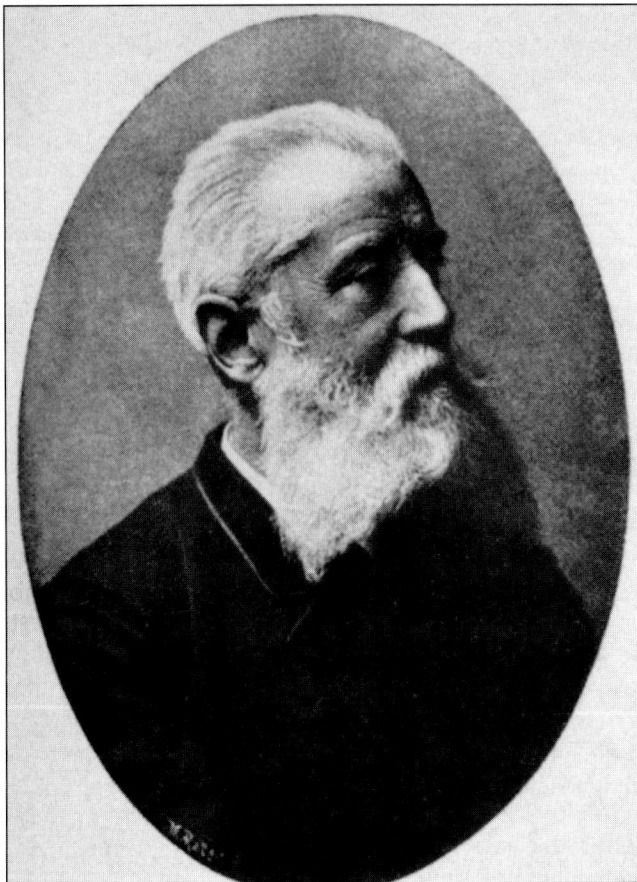

Figure 1.6 Friederich August von Esmarch. Reproduced by kind permission of the President and Council of the Royal College of Surgeons of England.

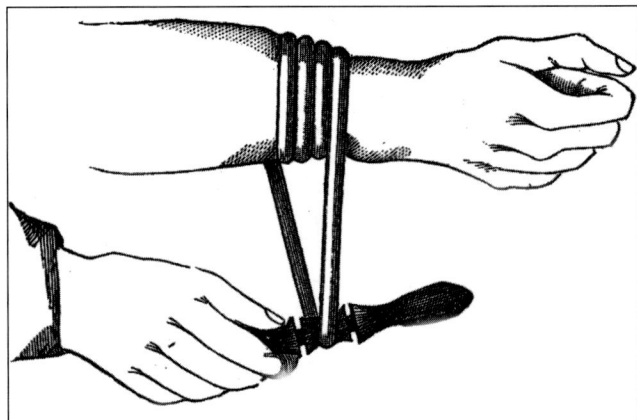

Figure 1.7 Application of Esmarch's bandage with a roller.

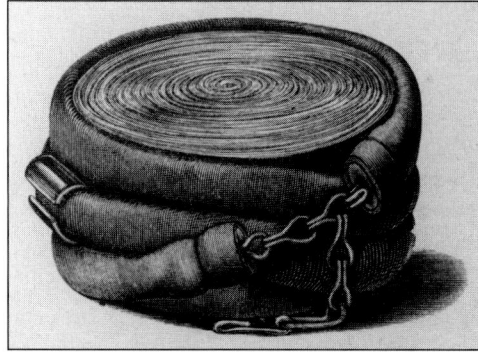

Figure 1.8 Esmarch (von Langenbeck) bandage with a rubber tourniquet. (a) Esmarch's apparatus for the bloodless operation.

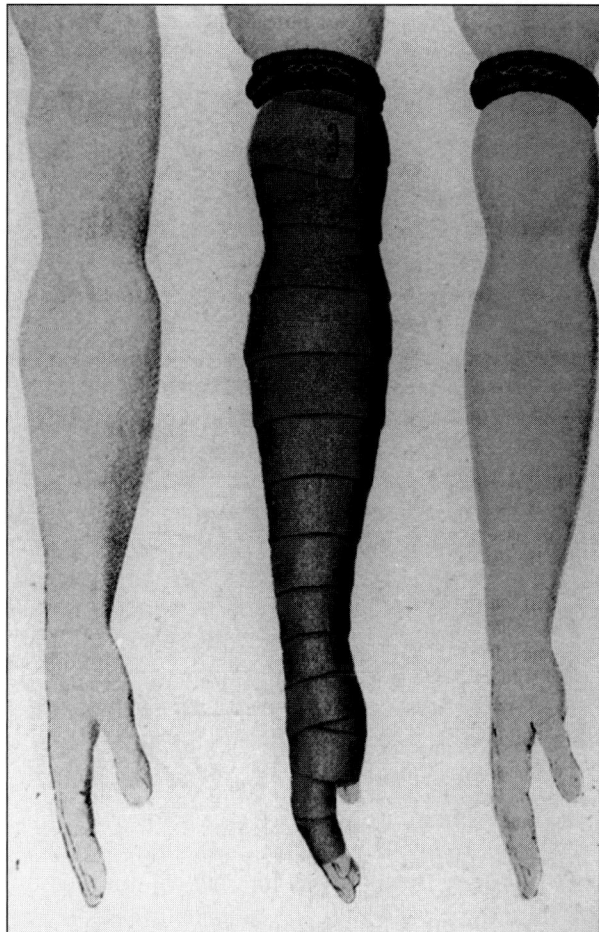

Figure 1.8 (b) Application of the tourniquet. Reproduced by kind permission of the President and Council of the Royal College of Surgeons of England.

4 When the elastic bandage is taken off . . . if the circulation has been effectively cut off the limb exhibits a completely blanched appearance like that of a dead subject, and any operation can be performed without loss of blood in dead subject.

Parts which contain unhealthy pus must not be firmly bandaged, for infecting matter may thereby be driven upwards into the cellular tissue, and into the lymphatics. In such cases one must be satisfied with raising the limb on high for a few minutes before applying the bandage, so as to diminish the amount of blood in the vessels.

Instead of a chain and hook, a clasp can be used for fixing the ends or a ligature employed through the cleft of which the stretched ends can be easily passed [Figure 1.8].

When Esmarch published his method of bloodless operation, Lister changed from using a Petit-type tourniquet to using Esmarch's rubber tourniquet, since the latter was more trustworthy and more convenient. Throughout his practice, however, he continued to empty a limb of blood by simple elevation.[5]

1.4 The Pneumatic Tourniquet

Harvey Cushing (Figure 1.9) introduced the pneumatic tourniquet to limb surgery in 1904.[11] He abandoned the rubber tourniquet because it carried the danger of nerve palsy: "out of a considerable number of pressure paralyses which have come under the writer's observation during the past two years, eight of them have thus originated ... the greater of these were of the brachial type".[11] In addition, the rubber tourniquet was difficult to remove and reapply rapidly during operation. The idea of an inflatable cuff originated from the use of the distensible armlet of the recently invented Riva-Rocci blood-pressure apparatus. As this armlet could be inflated only slowly, it allowed the limb to become engorged with blood before finally rendering it ischaemic; this made dissection difficult. Cushing then designed "a similar armlet, though broader, of less distensible rubber and of such quality that it would stand boiling ... and by connecting it with a bicycle pump of sufficient size one or two quick strokes of the piston sufficed to fill it".[11] As a refinement, he suggested inserting a manometer in the tube connecting the tourniquet pump and a tank of compressed air to maintain the required pressure. Cushing also used a pneumatic tourniquet as a constricting band about the head to prevent loss of blood while a skull flap was being raised. He later came to use a form of rubber ring in which a buckle was inserted so that a tube could be made into a ring of any size and could easily be removed at the end of the operation.

In his year abroad in 1900–1901, Cushing visited the Ospidale di S. Matteo clinic in Pavia, Italy. There, he found a simple "home-made" adaptation of Riva-Rocci's blood-pressure device, which was in daily routine use throughout the hospital. Cushing sketched this device and was given a model of the inflatable armlet, which he took back to Baltimore. Cushing and George Washington Crile were the first to advocate monitoring blood pressure during operations, and they introduced the first monitoring device into the theatre.[12]

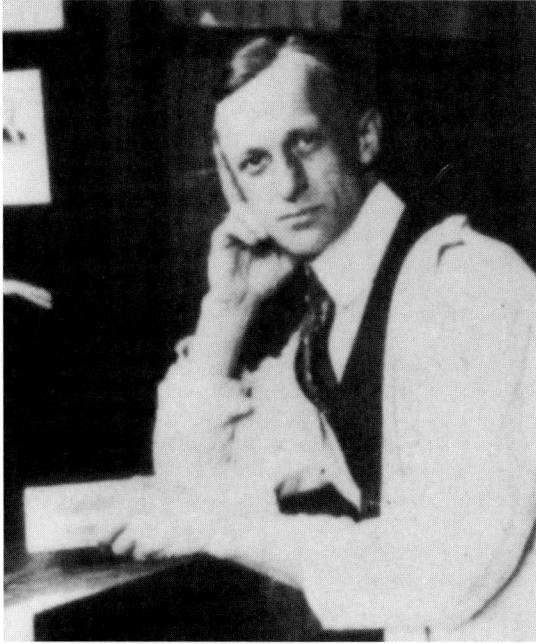

Figure 1.9 Harvey Cushing. Reproduced with permission from Fulton, J (1946). *Harvey Cushing.* Oxford: London.

Nowadays, it is routine practice to always use pneumatic tourniquets to obtain a bloodless field. These are found in increasing states of sophistication in all modern operating theatres and will be described in detail later in this text. The effects of the tourniquet on the tissues of the limb have been studied both clinically and experimentally in animals and form the basis of the following chapters.

References

1 Adams, F (1849). *The Genuine Works of Hippocrates.* Baltimore: Williams & Wilkins, p. 259.
2 Johnson, T (1649). *The Workes of that Famous Chirurgion Ambrose Parey.* London: Richard Cotes and Willi Du-gard, p. 339.
3 Yonge, J (1679). *Currus Triumphalis e Terebintho.* London: J. Martyn.
4 Chelius, JM (1847). *System of Surgery,* Vol. 1. London: Henry Renshaw.
5 Thompson, CJS (1942). *The History and Evolution of Surgical Instruments.* New York: Schuman's, p. 85.
6 Godlee, RJ (1924). *Lord Lister,* 3rd edn. Oxford: Clarendon Press, p. 632.
7 Lister, J (1909). *Collected Papers,* Vol. 1. Oxford: Clarendon Press, p. 176.
8 Von Esmarch, JFA (1873). Ueberkunstliche Blutleere bei Operationen. *Sammlung Klinischer Vorträge in Verbindung mit Deutschen Klinikern. Chirurgie* **58**(19): 373–384.
9 Fletcher, IR, Healy, TEJ (1983). The arterial tourniquet. *Annals of the Royal College of Surgeons* **65**: 410–417.
10 Von Esmarch, JFA (1878), transl. HH Clutton. *The Surgeon's Handbook on the Treatment of Wounded in War.* London: Sampson Low, Marston, Searle & Rivington, p. 127.
11 Cushing, H (1904). Pneumatic tourniquets: with especial reference to their use in craniotomies. *Medical News* **84**: 577–580.
12 Wangensteen OH, Wangensteen SD. *The Rise of Surgery.* Folkestone: William Dawson & Sons.

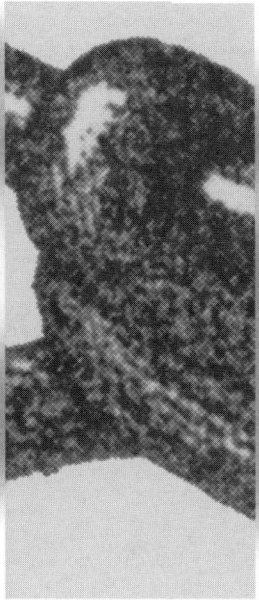

Chapter 2
**Effect of a Tourniquet on the Limb
and the Systemic Circulation**

THE DEPRIVATION OF blood, although temporary, tests the reserves of a limb, and it is important to use the tourniquet with discretion so that no permanent damage occurs. Essentially, a tourniquet should be applied only to limbs with normal blood supply. The effects of a tourniquet must be considered:

- on the tissues beneath the cuff, where there is both compression and ischaemia;
- distal to the cuff, where the effect is of ischaemia alone;
- on the systemic circulation.

2.1 Application of the Tourniquet

According to the American Heart Association, for accurate measurement of the blood pressure in the arm, the inflatable bag surrounded by an unyielding covering called the cuff must be the correct width for the diameter of the patient's arm.[1] If it is too narrow, the blood-pressure reading will be erroneously high; if it is too wide, the reading will be too low (Figure 2.1). The inflatable bag should be 20% wider than the diameter of the limb on which it is used. For an average adult, a bag of width 12–14 cm has been found to be satisfactory. The inflatable bag should be long enough to go halfway around the limb if care is taken to put the bag over the compressible artery. A bag of length 30 cm that nearly or completely encircles the limb obviates the risk of misapplication.

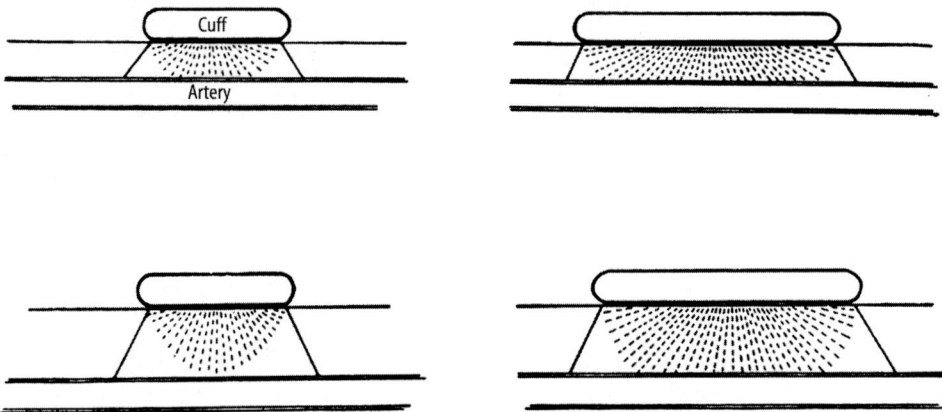

Figure 2.1 Diagram to show the difference in the transmission of pressure from a narrow cuff and a wide cuff to limbs of varying thickness.

The cuff should be made of non-distensible material so that, as far as possible, an even pressure is exerted throughout the cuff. Modern cuffs have fasteners that make it unnecessary to wrap a long cuff around the limb. Blood pressure in the thigh is measured by an 18–20-cm bag and an appropriately larger cuff. Although there is no consensus about the exact cuff size for thighs of different diameters and shapes, it is important that the cuff is wider and longer than that for the arm, in order to allow for the greater girth.

Standard, straight tourniquet cuffs are designed to fit optimally on cylindrically shaped limbs. However, sometimes limbs are conical in shape, especially in very muscular or obese individuals. Curved tourniquet cuffs have been designed for conical limbs and are more effective than straight cuffs at lower pressures in such limbs (Figure 2.2).[2]

Comparison of intra-arterial blood pressure in the arms and legs in humans shows that the femoral systolic blood pressure is approximately the same as that in the brachial artery.

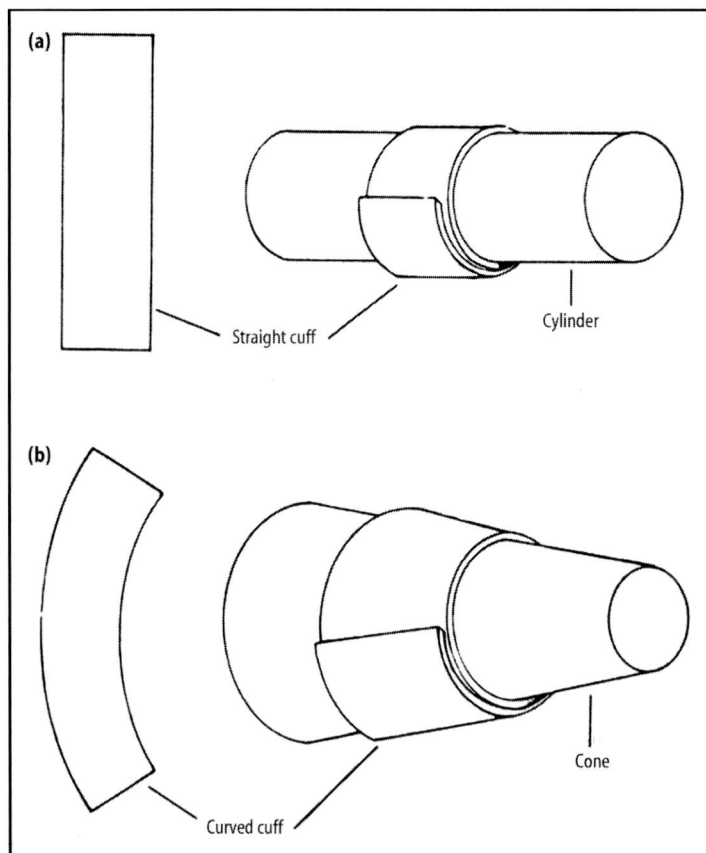

Figure 2.2 Schematic representation of (a) a straight tourniquet and (b) a curved tourniquet. Straight tourniquets fit optimally on cylindrical limbs, while curved tourniquets are designed to fit conical limbs.
Reprinted with permission of Lippincott, Williams & Wilkins from Pedowitz, RA, Gershuni, DH, Botte, MJ, et al. (1993). The use of lower tourniquet inflation pressures in extremity surgery facilitated by curved and wide tourniquets and an integrated cuff inflation system. *Clinical Orthopaedics and Related Research* 287: 237–243.

The principles for cuffs used as sphygmomanometers are also applicable to cuffs used as tourniquets, although allowances must be made for the situation in the operating theatre. Fluctuations of blood pressure may occur due to operative trauma; for the upper limb, an additional pressure of 50–75 mm Hg above systolic pressure (limb occlusion pressure) should be sufficient to prevent bleeding at the operation site. In the thigh, higher pressures are needed (Table 2.1): since the girth of the thigh is large and there is a need to keep well clear of the field of operation, the cuffs are narrower than those used to measure blood pressure. A simple rule of thumb in the thigh is to use double the systolic pressure in the arm.[3] This does not apply to children, for whom lower pressures can be used.[4]

Measurements on five cadaveric lower limbs were made directly beneath an 8.5-cm Kidde tourniquet cuff to establish the relationship beneath the pressure exerted by the tourniquet and that transmitted to the underlying soft tissues. The tissue pressure was consistently lower than the tourniquet pressure. The percentage of transmitted tourniquet pressure varied inversely with the circumference of the thigh.[5] There is a tendency for the soft-tissue pressure beneath a tourniquet cuff to decrease with the depth of soft tissue. This is minimal but becomes more pronounced as the circumference of the limb increases (Figure 2.3).

A tourniquet pressure of more than 300–350 mm Hg should rarely be required in normotensive individuals of normal habitus with compliant vessels. With the use of wide cuffs, the limb circumference is a determining factor in the transmission of pressure to the deep tissues. A cuff that is as wide as possible and is compatible with the surgical exposure should be used. Neimkin and Smith recommended using two tourniquet cuffs inflated alternately at hourly intervals without a reperfusion period; this avoided prolonged compression under the cuff.[6]

In another trial, tourniquet cuffs with widths varying from 4.5 to 80 cm were applied to the upper and lower extremities of 34 healthy, normotensive volunteers. Occlusion pressure was estimated by determining the level of cuff inflation at which the distal pulse became detectable by Doppler flow measurement. The occlusion pressure was

Table 2.1 Posterior tibial pressure measured using Doppler ultrasound and lower-calf tourniquet, and pressure of thigh tourniquet when Doppler signal has disappeared (occluding pressure). These measurements suggest that the commonly used pressure of 500 mm Hg (66.5 kPa) on the adult thigh is too high.

Sex of patient	Age (years)	Pedal pressure (posterior tibial) (mm Hg)*		Occluding pressure in thigh (mm Hg)*	
		Right	Left	Right	Left
Male	22	150	150	240	230
Female	26	160	160	200	200
Female	21	130	130	160	160
Female	38	130	130	180	190
Female	20	130	130	170	160
Female	23	130	130	180	190
Male	28	150	150	180	190
Female	25	155	160	200	200
Female	28	130	130	170	170

1 mm Hg ≈ 0.133 kPa.

Reprinted with permission from Klenerman, L (1978). A modified tourniquet. Journal of the Royal Society of Medicine 71: 121–122.

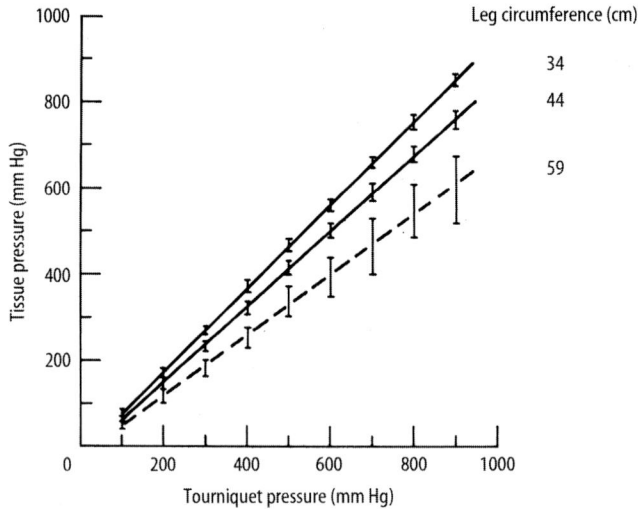

Figure 2.3 Mean soft-tissue pressure as a function of applied tourniquet pressure for thighs of different circumference. The vertical bars represent differences between the subcutaneous pressure and the pressure adjacent to the bone. Values for a 46-cm thigh are not shown in order to increase the clarity of the graph and avoid overlapping, but they were consistent with the pattern shown. Reproduced with permission from Shaw, JA, Murray, DG (1982). The relationship between tourniquet pressure and underlying soft tissue pressure in the thigh. *Journal of Bone and Joint Surgery* 64A: 1148–1151.

inversely proportional to the ratio of tourniquet cuff width to limb circumference. It was in a subsystolic range at a ratio above 0.5. The manner in which arterial flow is impeded by a wide tourniquet inflated to subsystolic pressure is not known. Accumulation of frictional resistance along a segment of a blood vessel that is partially collapsed under a low-pressure pneumatic tourniquet may completely eliminate flow without actual occlusion of the lumen region under the inflated cuff.[7]

Under the inflated cuff, there is a distribution of tissue from compressed to non-compressed zones, which includes mechanical deformation of all underlying tissues including muscles and nerve. This deformation is greatest under the edges of the cuff. Thus, the pressure gradient that is greatest at the edge of the compressed segment is the key factor in the occurrence of injuries to underlying tissues. Experimental studies confirm that muscle and nerve exhibit the most severe injuries at the upper and lower edges of the tourniquet cuff.[8] In experiments in which tourniquets were applied to the thighs of rabbits, the proximal border of the tourniquet induced severe vascular damage contributing to a "no-reflow phenomenon" in the muscle.[9]

2.2 Sites of Application

It has generally been considered that it is safest to apply a tourniquet to the proximal part of the limb, where the bulk of soft tissue provides the best protection for the underlying nerves and vessels. In addition, it was thought that a tourniquet applied to the forearm or calf might predispose to compartment syndrome. Recent reports have shown that this is not correct. Yousif and colleagues concluded that patients tolerate tourniquets on the upper arm and forearm equally well.[10] Hutchinson and McClintock found that in volunteers, tourniquets were tolerated for 44 minutes on the forearm and for 31 minutes on the upper arm.[11]

In a randomised, prospective trial on the position of the tourniquet on either the upper arm or the forearm in patients with carpal-tunnel decompression, both groups of patients tolerated the tourniquet equally well. However, the surgeons had some difficulty with the tourniquet on the forearm, as the patient's fingers may curl up and the tourniquet may be in the way when operating.[12] The authors concluded that there are very few indications for placing the tourniquet on the forearm in clinical practice.

A study of the use of a proximal calf tourniquet in 446 patients who had surgery on the foot and ankle showed that there were no complications to nerves or vessels.[13] The mean tourniquet time was 49.2 minutes for a single application and 131.1 minutes if there were two periods of tourniquet ischaemia. A tourniquet applied to the supramalleolar region of the leg has also been shown to be safe for surgery on the foot. The pressure was 100–150 mm Hg above systolic pressure and did not exceed 325 mm Hg. There were no complications. An ankle tourniquet with a regional ankle block provides a reasonable alternative to the standard thigh tourniquet for surgery of the foot.[14] For forefoot surgery, it has been shown that patients with an ankle tourniquet had significantly less pain during the operation than patients with a tourniquet on the calf, probably because of the smaller bulk of non-anaesthetised tissue.[15] Calf tourniquets are thus suitable only for hindfoot surgery.

2.3 Effect on Muscle

With the tourniquet in place in both animal models and human studies, oxygen tension and concentrations of creatine phosphate, glycogen and adenosine triphosphate (ATP) in muscle cells decrease with time, whereas carbon dioxide tension and lactate concentration increase as anaerobic metabolism occurs. Intracellular pH remains constant for 15 minutes, followed by a linear decrease to 6.0 after four hours of ischaemia. Intracellular creatine phosphate and ATP are depleted after two and three hours of ischaemia, respectively.[16]

Following the release of a tourniquet after two to four hours of ischaemia, an increase in microvascular permeability in muscle and nerve (demonstrated by the extravasation of Evans blue dye in animal studies) occurs as a result of both direct microvascular injury from compression and endothelial injury from superoxide radicals. Animal studies have also shown that after prolonged use of a tourniquet, there is a marked decrease in the production of force in muscles beneath and distal to the tourniquet (21–70% of control values).

Nevertheless, during tourniquet ischaemia, the muscle is at rest and the only expenditure of energy is for basal metabolism. Thus, in spite of the circulatory arrest, the biochemical changes are relatively slow.

2.3.1 Safe Period

The length of time that it is safe to leave a tourniquet in place on a healthy limb without causing irreversible damage to the skeletal muscle is of importance in orthopaedic practice. Present-day recommendations, based mainly on personal experience, vary from one hour (the opinion of Bruner in 1951),[17] to two hours (according to Boyes in 1964),[18] with an upper limit of three hours (according to Parkes in 1973).[19] Compression and ischaemia are the factors most likely to contribute to the muscular damage. Changes in the muscle resulting from tourniquet-induced ischaemia have been studied from many aspects, including histological,[20] histo-chemical,[21] biochemical[22] and ultrastructural.[23–25] However, the effect of compression on the muscle lying immediately under the tourniquet has received little attention.

2.3.2 Effects on the Ultrastructure of Muscle

Mammalian muscle is composed of three main types of fibre: fast-twitch white, fast-twitch red, and slow-twitch intermediate.[25] The fast-twitch red and slow-twitch intermediate fibres rely primarily on oxidative metabolism and are more resistant to fatigue than the mainly glycolytic fast-twitch white fibres.

Using the soleus and the extensor digitorum longus, which between them contain representatives of all three types of fibre, the possibility of a differential response to ischaemia was investigated in adult rhesus monkeys weighing 3.5–5 kg.[26] Under anaesthesia, a Kidde tourniquet cuff of infant size was applied to the upper thigh of the right lower limb for periods lasting from one to five hours at a pressure of 300 mm Hg. Immediately before the release of the tourniquet, samples from the soleus and the extensor digitorum longus were removed for biopsy and processed for electron microscopy. Samples from the muscle lying under the tourniquet, the quadriceps, were taken after removal of the tourniquet.

Recovery from three-hour and five-hour tourniquets was investigated. Samples from the quadriceps, extensor digitorum longus and soleus were taken one day, two or three days, and seven days after release of the tourniquet. Only one sample was removed from any one particular muscle since, in trial experiments, repeated sampling was found to cause marked damage to the fibres. Samples from the opposite limb were used as controls. The specimens were examined using electron microscopy (Figure 2.4).

2.3.3 Effects of Ischaemia on Muscles Distal to the Tourniquet

In the experiment described in the previous section, after one hour of ischaemia marked changes in mitochondrial morphology were observed in the fibres of both the extensor digitorum longus and the soleus. The fibres had become swollen and less electron-dense, and they had lost their organised network of cristae, although many fibres displaying normal mitochondrial morphology were still present. As the period of ischaemia was increased progressively up to five hours, a greater percentage of the fibres showed mitochondrial damage, which was similar in all three types of fibre (Figure 2.5). Except for a reduction in the number of granules of glycogen in the fast-twitch red and fast-twitch white fibres, ischaemia had no immediate effect on any other component of the fibres.

Recovery of the extensor digitorum longus and the soleus from a three-hour tourniquet was rapid. One day after release of the tourniquet, the majority of fibres in both muscles appeared normal. Fibres with spaces, usually at the level of the I-band, were encountered occasionally. Frequently, these spaces contained membranous material, which probably represented the remains of degenerating mitochondria. The levels of glycogen returned to those found in control fibres.

A similar result was obtained in the soleus one day after a five-hour tourniquet, but in the extensor digitorum longus infiltrating polymorphs and damaged and normal fibres were found. The damaged fibres had enlarged mitochondria, the Z-discs were eroded away, and electron-dense deposits were found interspersed between the myofibrils. Except for a few fibres containing the remnants of degenerating mitochondria, the majority of fibres from both muscles recovered totally three days after a five-hour tourniquet. The extensive damage found in the extensor digitorum longus one day after a five-hour tourniquet was not observed in any of the fibres examined. After seven days, all the fibres that had been subjected to a five-hour period of ischaemia were indistinguishable from those of the control muscles.

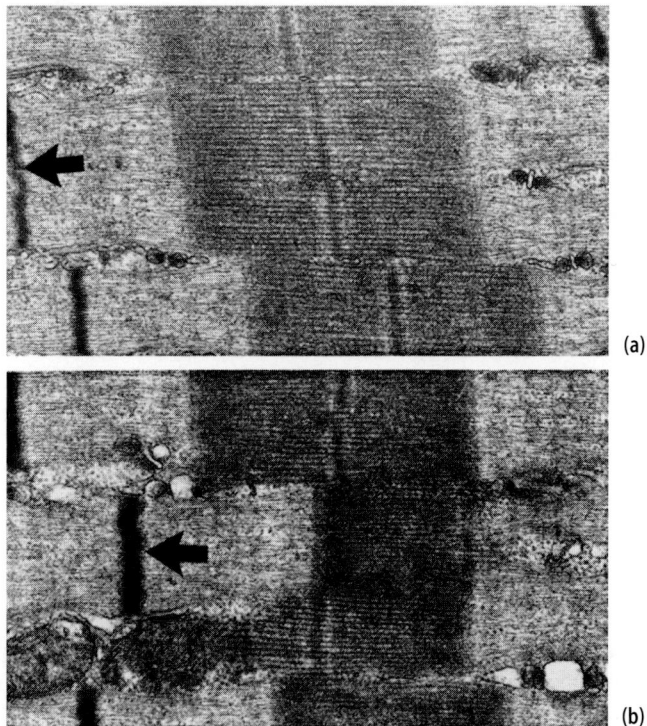

(a)

(b)

Figure 2.4 Longitudinal section through normal extensor digitorum longus. Note the difference in thickness between the Z-discs of (a) the fast-twitch white fibre (arrow) and (b) the fast-twitch red fibre (arrow) (×30 800). Reprinted with permission from Patterson, S, Klenerman, L (1979). The effect of pneumatic tourniquets on the ultrastructure of skeletal muscle. *Journal of Bone and Joint Surgery* 61B: 178–183.

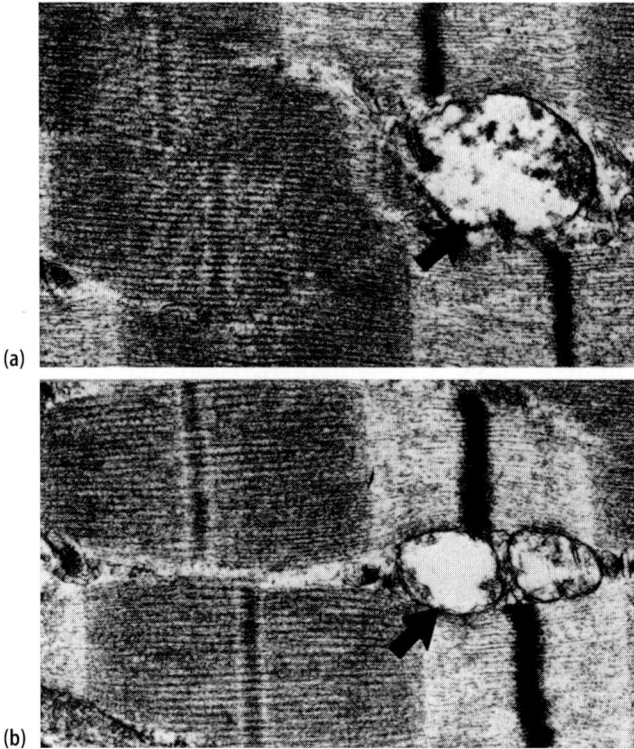

(a)

(b)

Figure 2.5 Longitudinal sections through soleus sampled immediately after an ischaemic period of three hours. Swollen mitochondria that have lost their organised array of cristae are present in both (a) the slow-twitch intermediate fibre (arrow) and (b) the fast-twitch red fibre (arrow) (×34 600). Reprinted with permission from Patterson, S, Klenerman, L (1979). The effect of pneumatic tourniquets on the ultrastructure of skeletal muscle. *Journal of Bone and Joint Surgery* 61B: 178–183.

2.3.4 Effects of Compression and Ischaemia in the Quadriceps

All samples both immediately and 24 hours after removal of the three-hour tourniquet were normal, except for a slight swelling of the mitochondria. In one experiment in which the muscle was examined two days after the release of the tourniquet, approximately 50% of the fibres showed significant changes. The I- and Z-bands were lost, and the remaining A-bands were frequently disoriented, so filaments sectioned in a longitudinal plane lay adjacent to others cut transversely. The mitochondria of these fibres often contained electron-dense products (Figures 2.6 and 2.7). Polymorphs were found in the interfibre spaces and sometimes penetrating between the myofibrils. All muscle fibres examined seven days after the release of the three-hour tourniquet were morphologically identical to those of control fibres.

Muscle samples from the quadriceps taken immediately after the release of the five-hour tourniquet showed extensive mitochondrial damage, similar to that observed in the ischaemic extensor digitorum longus and soleus. In addition, there was slight filament erosion at the Z- and I-band levels, and the sarcolemma was broken and fragmented. One day after release of the tourniquet, the Z-disc was totally eroded from all the fibres examined. The thin actin filaments no longer appeared rigid and straight but ran a spidery path into the A-band. The mitochondria remained swollen and pale, and the sarcolemma was fragmented. Polymorphs and red cells were frequently found in the interfibre spaces.

On the third day after release of the five-hour tourniquet, many totally necrotic fibres were found. These fibres were filled with amorphous material and did not show the characteristic areas of A-, I- and Z-bands (Figure 2.8). Fibres with intact filament and triad systems were also common at this stage of recovery. However, such fibres often contained large myelin figures (Figure 2.9). Fibroblast cells lying between the fibres were encountered occasionally.

Approximately two-thirds of the fibres had intact contractile filament and triad systems seven days after the release of the five-hour tourniquet. Dense amorphous material was found lying between the myofibrils in a small number of these fibres. The remaining fibres appeared to be engaged in resynthesising contractile material. The nuclei of these fibres often occupied a more central position, and stretches of endoplasmic reticulum were dispersed throughout their cytoplasm.

Tourniquets applied for long periods caused more severe and lasting damage to the muscle lying beneath the tourniquet than the muscles lying distal to it. The sarcolemmal damage observed in fibres of the quadriceps immediately after removal of a five-hour tourniquet would have detrimental effects on their excitation–contraction coupling system. The total erosion of the Z-discs found 24 hours after removal of a five-hour tourniquet would render the development of tension impossible in these fibres.

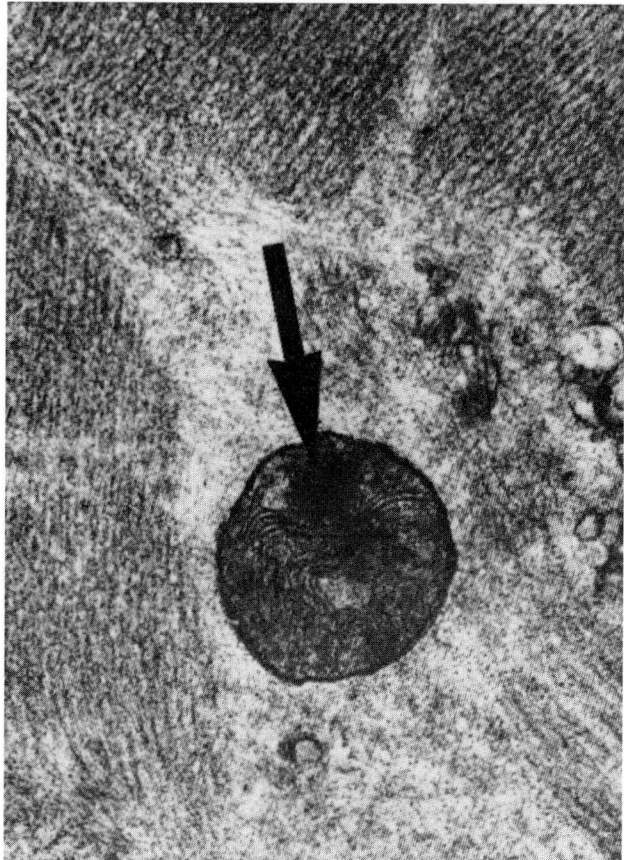

Figure 2.6 Transverse section through the quadriceps two days after release of a three-hour tourniquet. The myofibrils are disoriented and electron-dense products are present in the mitochondria (arrow) ($\times$30 800). Reprinted with permission from Patterson, S, Klenerman, L (1979). The effect of pneumatic tourniquets on the ultrastructure of skeletal muscle. *Journal of Bone and Joint Surgery* 61B: 178–183.

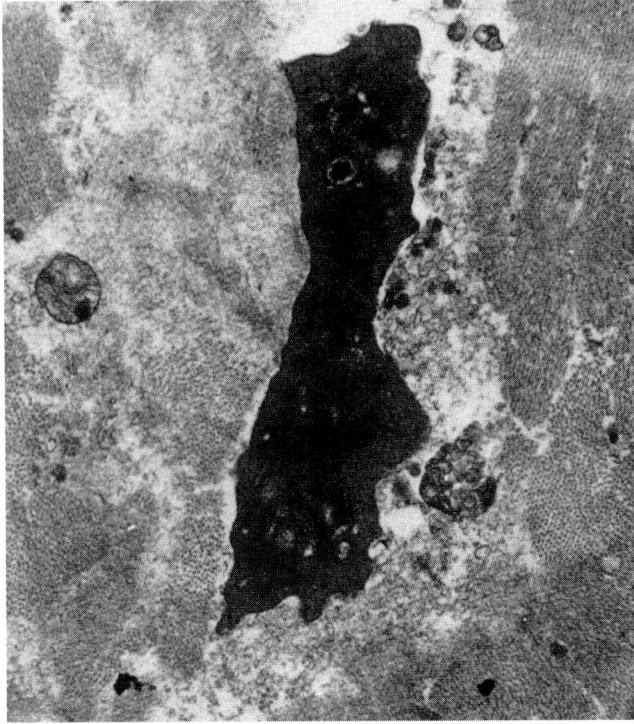

Figure 2.7 Section through myofibrils of muscle. A polymorph can be seen penetrating the myofibrils (×12 800). Reprinted with permission from Patterson, S, Klenerman, L (1979). The effect of pneumatic tourniquets on the ultrastructure of skeletal muscle. *Journal of Bone and Joint Surgery* 61B: 178–183.

Although fibres with a reasonably normal structure were found on the third and seventh days after the release of a five-hour tourniquet, the general ultrastructural picture was still aberrant. Even fibres with intact contractile systems were occasionally found to have deposits of amorphous material lying between the myofibrils. The nature of this amorphous material is not known.

The duration for which a tourniquet is left in place appears to be a critical factor in determining whether severe damage occurs to the underlying muscle. After five hours, there was evidence of severe damage in all the muscle samples examined subsequently. On the other hand, only one of four monkeys showed any sign of severe damage after the use of a three-hour tourniquet. It may be that three hours is close to the limit of time that a muscle can resist sustained compression and that the muscles of more susceptible individuals succumb after this period. Although a number of investigators have reported the effect of ischaemia on muscles distal to the tourniquet, their findings have not always been uniform. There is general agreement that the mitochondria swell and the cristae become disorganised. Tountas and Bergman, working with cynomologus monkeys, found that the mitochondria were the only components of the muscle fibre to undergo change, and seven days after the release of the tourniquet the muscle was normal.[23] Dissolution of the Z-discs was observed 16 hours after two-hour tourniquets were released from the limbs of mice.[22] In studies in the rabbit, tourniquets applied for little as 30 minutes resulted in degenerating fibres and infiltrating phagocytic cells, visible with the light microscope, being found one day later.[21]

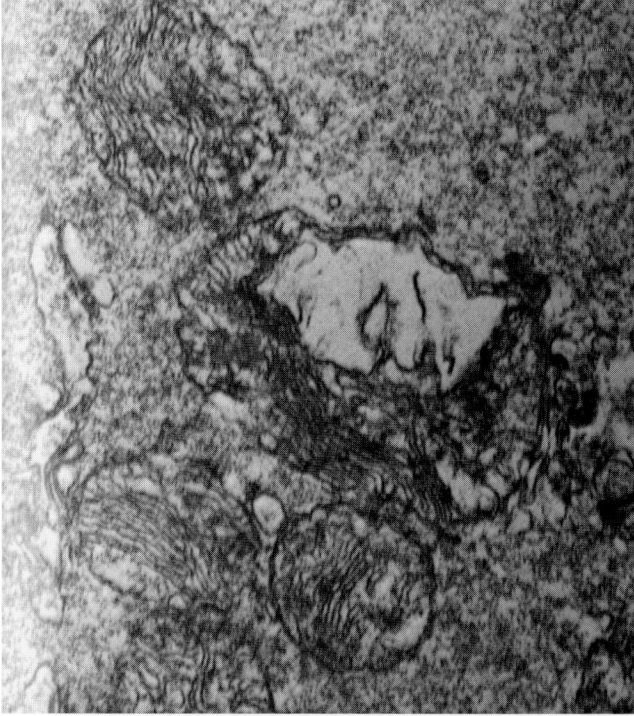

Figure 2.8 Transverse section of the quadriceps three days after the release of a five-hour tourniquet. This fibre has totally lost its characteristic areas of A-, I- and Z-bands (×30 800). Reprinted with permission from Patterson, S, Klenerman, L (1979). The effect of pneumatic tourniquets on the ultrastructure of skeletal muscle. *Journal of Bone and Joint Surgery* 61B: 178–183.

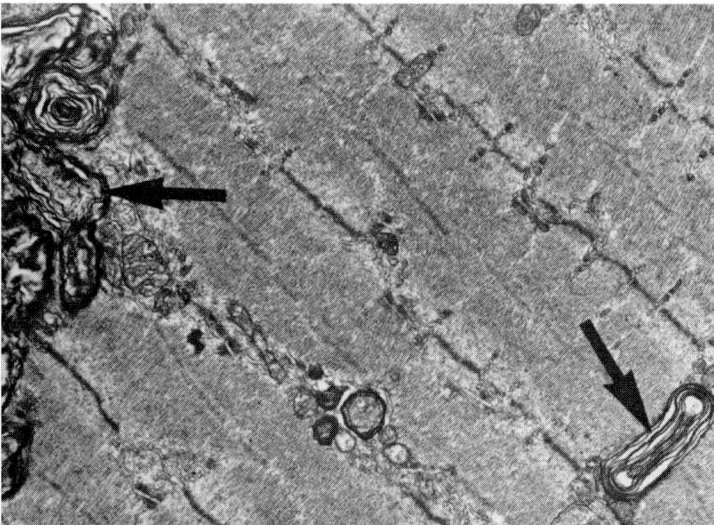

Figure 2.9 Longitudinal section through the quadriceps three days after the release of a five-hour tourniquet. The contractile filament system is intact but large myelin figures are present (arrows) (×9600). Reprinted with permission from Patterson, S, Klenerman, L (1979). The effect of pneumatic tourniquets on the ultrastructure of skeletal muscle. *Journal of Bone and Joint Surgery* 61B: 178–183.

In the experiments with rhesus monkeys, the mitochondria were the only components of the extensor digitorum longus and soleus to show any significant degree of damage after a three-hour tourniquet. These organelles seem to be very sensitive to ischaemia, since changes were observed after only one hour. In studies on ischaemic heart muscle, mitochondrial damage was observed after as little as 12 minutes.27 The soleus and extensor digitorum longus of the rhesus monkeys showed a remarkable ability to regenerate their mitochondria. Mitochondrial structure was normal three days after a three-hour period of ischaemia and seven days after five hours of ischaemia. It was interesting to find normal fibres interspersed with others showing mitochondrial damage. Moore and colleagues22 reported similar observations in ischaemic muscle in mice.

Resistance or susceptibility of the mitochondria of muscle fibre to ischaemia does not appear to be related to the type of fibre, since similar changes were observed in all three types. The metabolism of fast-twitch red and slow-twitch intermediate fibres is primarily oxidative, while the fast-twitch white fibres are mainly glycolytic. Physiologically, this may be manifested in the former two types giving earlier fatigue times.

The more severe effects of ischaemia observed by some workers may be related to the species of animal studied. In the rhesus monkey, a three-hour tourniquet did not result in damage to the contractile filaments. However, in one monkey subjected to a five-hour tourniquet, infiltrating cells and eroded Z-discs were found in the extensor digitorum longus one day after tourniquet release. This may indicate that five hours of ischaemia is close to the limit of time that the muscle can endure ischaemia without becoming severely damaged.

Histologically, the contractile machinery of the muscle fibres of the rhesus monkey appeared to be wholly unaffected by periods of ischaemia lasting up to three hours. However, from the functional aspect, this was not so. Tests for strength in cynomologus monkeys after three- or five-hour tourniquets using infant-size Kidde cuffs were carried out.28 Development of maximum isometric tension, contraction times and half-relaxation times were measured in the muscles beneath and distal to the tourniquet. On release of the tourniquet, no consistent difference between control and experimental muscles was observed with respect to contraction and half-relaxation times; however, there was a marked reduction in the development of isometric tension. On the sixth day after release of a five-hour tourniquet, isometric tension was reduced to 2–22% of the control value of the compressed muscle. Six days after a three-hour tourniquet, isometric tension of the compressed muscle was 80% of control value; in the distal gastrocnemius–soleus complex, tension varied from 64% to control value. It is clear that the effect on muscle contraction after a three-hour period of ischaemia is not reversed immediately by restoration of the blood supply. It is surprising that the reduction in isometric tension was greater in the gastrocnemius–soleus complex than in the compressed quadriceps muscle. A possible explanation for this is the morphology of the muscle. The fibres do not all run the whole length of the quadriceps as the rectus femoris is bipennate. As the tourniquet cuff was in the middle of the thigh, it is possible that this resulted in a mixed effect on contractile power.

Similar experiments on New Zealand white rabbits showed that tourniquet compression for two hours resulted in markedly reduced force production beneath and also distal to the tourniquet cuff. Two days after compression, maximal quadriceps force production was reduced to 40% of control values with 125 mm Hg compression and to 21% of control values after 350 mm Hg compression. The maximal force production of the tibialis anterior declined to 70% and 24%, respectively.[29] Although tissues distal to the tourniquet were usually accepted as affected by ischaemia alone, these workers considered that proximal compression of the nerve supply to the tibialis anterior beneath the tourniquet had interfered with nerve function.

In summary, the experiments on rhesus monkeys have shown more marked changes in the muscles beneath the cuff than those distal to the cuff. Three hours seems to be close to the time limit for the safe application of a tourniquet because of the combined effects of compression and ischaemia on the muscle beneath the cuff.

2.3.5 No-reflow Phenomenon

Attempts at reperfusion may not always be successful because of progressive microcirculatory obstruction. This process, called the "no-reflow phenomenon", is related to the length of the ischaemic interval. Muscles that have been ischaemic for one to three hours are easily reperfused, but the no-reflow phenomenon occurs in 40–50% of cases after five hours of ischaemia.[30] The exact cause is not understood fully. Microscopy has shown large numbers of red cells in the microcirculation. Cellular oedema may also lead to capillary plugging during reperfusion.[31]

2.3.6 Effect on the Function of the Underlying Quadriceps Muscle

It has been assumed that movement of the muscle is restricted by an inflated tourniquet. An investigation was carried out in five healthy male volunteers using ultrasound to measure the movement of the quadriceps muscle above and below the tourniquet, before and after inflation.[32] A tourniquet of standard size was applied to the thigh for five minutes. A bubble of air was injected into the muscle above the tourniquet and was the proximal point of reference. The musculotendinous junction was the distal point. The movement of the reference point was measured by ultrasound before and after each inflation of the tourniquet. Each measurement was repeated with either the knee flexed and the hip extended, or the hip flexed and the knee extended. The ultrasound findings consistently showed no evidence of restriction of the quadriceps muscle by an inflated tourniquet. The authors recommend that the tourniquet be inflated in the most convenient position for the surgeon.

2.4 Compression of Nerves

According to Lundborg, inflation of a cuff to suprasystolic pressure around the arm results in a conduction block, rapidly reversible upon the release of the cuff.[9]

Pressure just sufficient to occlude the underlying blood vessels results in a block of nerve conduction in 15–45 minutes. At a cuff pressure of 150 mm Hg, sensory loss and paralysis develop at the same rate as when a pressure of 300 mm Hg is used. This indicates that ischaemia rather than mechanical pressure is the underlying cause of such conduction block, which is rapidly reversible and physiological. When the cuff is inflated to a higher pressure, there is a risk of mechanical damage to the nerve fibres, resulting in a longer-lasting conduction block – a local demyelinating block, which has been called "tourniquet paralysis".[33, 34] The underlying force seems to be the pressure gradient within the nerve between its compressed and uncompressed portions, the displacements being away from the region of high pressure towards the uncompressed region beyond the edge of the cuff tourniquet.

The biological basis of localised conduction blocks induced by direct pressure has been analysed extensively in a series of experimental studies.[33–35] These experiments were carried out on baboons, with a tourniquet cuff pressure of about 1000 mm Hg for 90–180 minutes. When single teased fibres were examined within a few hours or days, they showed a specific morphological phenomenon: under each border zone of the compressed segment, the nodes of Ranvier had been displaced along each fibre, so that the paranodal myelin was stretched on one side of the node and invaginated on the other. The whole picture is strongly reminiscent of an intussusception, as it occurs in the bowel. The underlying force seemed to be the pressure gradient within the nerve between its compressed and uncompressed portions. In each case, the displacement was away from the region of high pressure towards the uncompressed region beyond the edge of the cuff (Figure 2.10).

The result was localised degenerative changes of the damaged myelin (paranodal demyelination). Only large myelinated fibres were affected. In these experiments, a cuff pressure of 1000 mm Hg maintained for one to three hours produced paralysis of distal muscles lasting for up to three months. There was a significant correlation between the duration of compression and the duration of the subsequent conduction block. The effects of the block correspond with the type of

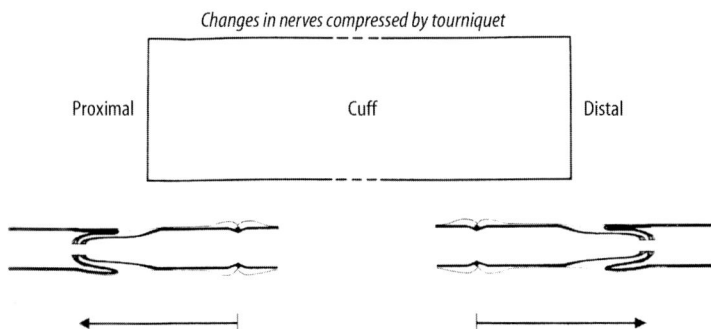

Changes in nerves compressed by tourniquet

Proximal   Cuff   Distal

Figure 2.10 Diagram to show the direction of displacement of nodes of Ranvier in relation to the cuff. Reprinted with permission from Ochoa, J, Fowler, TJ, Gilliatt, RW (1972). Anatomical changes in peripheral nerves compressed by a pneumatic tourniquet. *Journal of Anatomy* 113: 433–455.

nerve injury classified by Seddon in 1943 as neuropraxia.[36] Gilliatt in 1980 showed by direct recordings from the exposed nerve "a double conduction block" affecting the large myelinated fibres as two separate regions of the nerve trunk corresponding in position to both edges of the cuff, while the intermediate region showed little or no change in conduction.[37]

2.5 Effects on the Skin

On the whole, the skin is resilient and unaffected in the vast majority of cases of tourniquet use. Damage at the site of the tourniquet may be caused by pressure necrosis or friction burns. Such burns are thought to be caused by spirit-based antiseptic solutions that seep beneath the tourniquet and are held against the skin under pressure (see Chapter 5).[38]

Friction burns may result during operations on the thigh due to a fully inflated tourniquet cuff slipping down and away from the plaster wool padding.[39] An investigation on the effects produced by commonly used antiseptic paints and a known chemical irritant, anthralin, was carried out on the upper arms and forearms of volunteers.[40] Site-related variations in anthralin-induced inflammation were observed, but there was no demonstrable effect of either pressure or ischaemia on the inflammatory response. It was not possible to keep the tourniquets in place for longer than half an hour because it would have been too painful for the volunteers to tolerate the pain of ischaemia. It was concluded that burns under tourniquets are likely to be idiosyncratic reactions, and their further investigation required detailed examination of individuals affected by chemical burns.

2.6 Systemic and Local Effects of the Application of a Tourniquet

There have been few reports describing the systemic effects of reperfusing the ischaemic limb.[41, 42] Complete arrest of the circulation to the limb produces acidosis and changes in levels of potassium,[43, 44] which in theory could result in effects on the rhythm of the heart when the tourniquet is released. Although changes in the acid–base status of the blood leaving the limb have been described, the state of the blood reaching the heart after the release of a tourniquet has received little attention.[45] An animal and clinical study was undertaken to establish whether any biochemical changes in the limb are reflected in the right atrium. In addition, the time taken for the ischaemic limb to recover was investigated.[46]

2.6.1 Animal Experiments

An infant-size Kidde tourniquet cuff 5 cm wide was applied to the experimental limb of a rhesus monkey and inflated to a pressure of 300 mm Hg for a predetermined

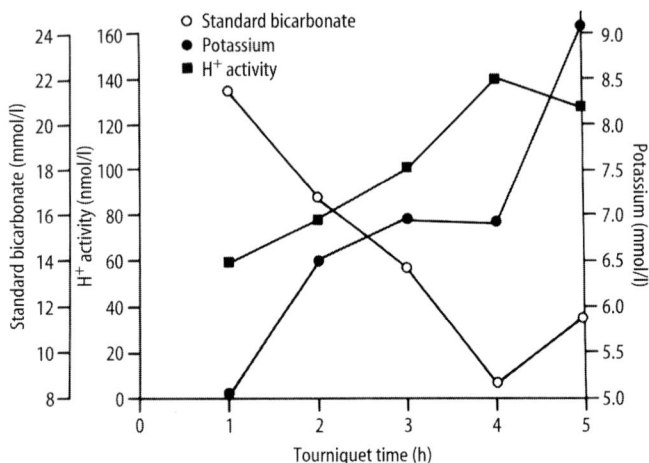

Figure 2.11 Mean initial readings from the first sample of blood from the limb after release of the tourniquet plotted against the time for which the tourniquet was inflated. Reprinted with permission from Klenerman, L, Biswas, M, Hulands, GH, Rhodes, AM (1980). Systemic and local effects of the application of a tourniquet. *Journal of Bone and Joint Surgery* 62B: 385–388.

time from one to five hours. At regular intervals during the period when the tourniquet was in place, samples were taken over a period of one minute from the cannula in the right atrium to establish control values for acid–base status and potassium levels. After the release of the tourniquet, further samples were taken simultaneously from both the internal jugular route and the femoral vein for periods as long as two hours.

Whenever possible, all samples were measured immediately for pCO_2, pH, excess of base, and standard bicarbonate. If this was not possible, samples were stored in ice for no longer than 30 minutes.

When the tourniquet was released, samples taken from the right side of the heart showed little or no change in acid–base status. The longer the tourniquet had been in place, the greater were the biochemical changes in the limb (Figure 2.11). The readings for pH, potassium and pCO_2 in the right atrium immediately before the release of the tourniquet were taken as 100%. Each subsequent reading taken from the atrium and the femoral vein was then expressed as a percentage of the initial reading.

The results obtained were plotted on semilogarithmic paper. The best-fit line for each variable was drawn for the samples for the heart and limb. Recovery time for the limb was measured at the point where the initial slope of the curve for the limb intersected with the line for readings from the right side of the heart. This was plotted against the time for which the tourniquet had been inflated (Figure 2.12). After one hour with the tourniquet, recovery occurred in the limb within 20 minutes. For tourniquet periods of two to four hours, recovery of all variables was complete with 40 minutes. However, after five hours of tourniquet use, recovery for potassium and standard bicarbonate occurred within one hour and 40 minutes, but pH returned to the level of the blood in the right atrium after two hours and 40 minutes.

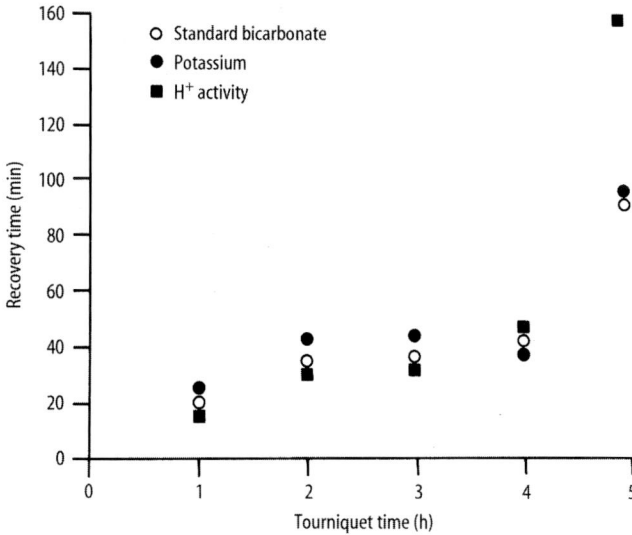

Figure 2.12 Estimated recovery time for each variable in the blood supply in the limb subjected to ischaemia in relation to the time for which the tourniquet was used.

Reprinted with permission from Klenerman, L, Biswas, M, Hulands, GH, Rhodes, AM (1980). Systemic and local effects of the application of a tourniquet. *Journal of Bone and Joint Surgery* 62B: 385–388.

2.6.2 Clinical Studies

Patients who were about to undergo total knee replacement or a high tibial osteotomy for rheumatoid arthritis or osteoarthritis were informed of the studies and consented to participate. All patients received appropriate premedication of papaveretum and atropine. Anaesthesia was induced with thiopentone, an intravenous injection of pancuronium was given, and intubation was carried out. Anaesthesia was maintained with nitrous oxide, oxygen and phenoperidine, and occasionally halothane (less than 0.5%). Ventilation was adjusted for a standard $paCO_2$ of 5.4 kPa. A cannula was passed via the right internal jugular vein into the atrium and its position checked by looking for atrial oscillations; 5% dextrose solution was infused. An intravenous drip of Hartmann's solution was set up in one forearm. The electrocardiogram was displayed continuously, and the temperature was monitored by a nasopharyngeal probe. An Esmarch bandage was used to exsanguinate the site of operation, and a 10-cm Kidde tourniquet cuff was inflated to occlude the arterial flow at a pressure of twice the pre-induction systolic pressure. During the operation, several samples were taken from the internal jugular cannula to establish baseline values for blood analysis from the central venous pool. At the end of the operation, pressure dressings were applied to the limb while the tourniquet was still inflated. Samples of blood were taken from the atrium via the internal jugular cannula and also from the femoral vein of the operated limb by direct needle stab just before releasing the tourniquet. When the tourniquet was released, samples were taken simultaneously from the femoral needle and the internal jugular cannula for a period of approximately 15 minutes and then intermittently from the jugular cannula for approximately two hours. These samples were analysed as described above.

There were nine patients (three men, six women), of average age 68 years (range 51–80 years). The tourniquet was inflated for periods ranging from 70 to 186 minutes.

2.6.3 Results of Investigations

There were only minor fluctuations in the three variables – potassium, bicarbonate and pH – in the samples taken from the right atrium. These transiently reflected the marked changes that occurred in the blood from the limb. No cardiac dysrhythmias were detected on monitoring.

Neither the patients nor the experimental animals showed evidence of nerve palsies.

In a limb that has been rendered ischaemic, metabolites accumulate as a result of hypoxia in the tissues. Theoretically, a rapid influx of some of these products, e.g. potassium, into the coronary circulation is likely to produce cardiac dysfunction. In these studies, although the potassium levels in the blood leaving the limb were raised, at no time was a significant rise detected in the right atrium either in the animals or in the patients. The most likely explanation for this is a dilutional effect due to the larger volume of blood contained in the venous side of the circulation (50% of the circulating blood volume is accommodated on the venous side, but only 15% is in the arterial system). Similarly, the fall in pH in the venous blood leaving the acidotic limb was not reflected in the acid–base status of the blood samples from the right atrium. Again, the effect of dilution is a factor here, but in addition there is the efficient buffering capacity of the blood. A criticism of the sampling technique used could be based on the well-known streaming effect of blood from the venae cavae. This is well documented in relation to the measurement of venous oxygen in estimations of cardiac output. However, the authors were not aware of work showing that this effect was also applicable to other biochemical measurements. Although streaming within the atrium cannot be discounted, it is unlikely to be an important factor as the results were consistent. These findings are essentially in agreement with those described in patients undergoing operations under tourniquet with lumbar epidural anaesthesia.[45]

In the animal studies, it was found that the acid–base balance in the limb returned to normal within 20 minutes of the release of a tourniquet that had been in place for one hour, and within 40 minutes after four hours of ischaemia. The practice of releasing the tourniquet at two hours for a period of five to ten minutes to allow a "breathing period" therefore does not seem appropriate.

The investigations that have been described were undertaken in healthy animals and fit patients who did not suffer from cardiovascular disease. When, as is not uncommon, the buffering capacity is reduced by anaemia, hypovolaemia, metabolic acidosis or pre-existing vascular disease, there is likely to be a reduction in the normal range of safety. In addition, under certain conditions a compromised myocardium may be sensitised to catecholamines by anaesthetic agents. In these circumstances, the period for which a tourniquet is used should be reduced to the minimum and full cardiovascular monitoring must be available. The changes noted in the acid–base balance indicate that a period of three hours under a tourniquet is safe. This coincides with findings made in histological studies of the ischaemic muscle.[26]

2.7 Haemodynamic Changes

The haemodynamic changes associated with the application and release of a tourniquet are minimal in healthy adults, but they may not be tolerated by patients with poor cardiac reserve. In a series of patients who were monitored for changes in central venous pressure (CVP) and systolic blood pressure, it was found that the main rise in CVP with the application of bilateral tourniquets was 14.5 cm H_2O.[47] This was maintained in 80% of patients until the tourniquets were released (Figure 2.13). It is likely that this was due to an increase of approximately 15% of circulating blood volume – about 700–800 ml of blood. In comparison, the CVP values when single tourniquets were applied showed that the circulation could deal with the smaller autotransfusion of blood more easily. The mean systolic pressure change was ±18.5 mm Hg when the tourniquets were inflated. On deflation, the mean fall below the blood pressure at the start of surgery was 43.5 mm Hg. The initial rise in blood pressure either was sustained or fell gradually to the level before a tourniquet was applied, and then had a further dramatic fall within three minutes of release of the tourniquet. In a review of the records of 500 patients who had surgery under a tourniquet, the frequency of intraoperative hypertension (defined as a 30% increase in either systolic or diastolic pressure compared with the first pressure recording after incision) was 11%. The probability of hypertension was increased if the patient was elderly, had cardiac enlargement as shown by X-ray or electrocardiogram (ECG), or had nitrous oxide and narcotic anaesthesia. Pre-existing hypertension, increased serum creatinine concentration, anaemia, or treatment with hypertensive drugs were not associated strongly with intraoperative hypertension.[48] Patients with head injuries and multiple sites of trauma may have marked increases in intracranial pressure when lower limb tourniquets are released.[49]

Using transoesophageal echocardiography during 59 total knee replacements, it was found that showers of echogenic material traversed the right atrium, right ventricle and pulmonary artery after the tourniquets were deflated.[50] This was observed in various degrees in all patients and lasted for 3–15 minutes. The mean peak intensity occurred within 30 seconds (range 24–45 seconds) after the tourniquet was released. Only three patients had evidence of clinical pulmonary embolism. These findings are similar to those described by Parmet and colleagues in a smaller series of 29 patients.[51] This group aspirated a 3 × 6-mm fresh thrombus from a central catheter in one patient. Another patient, who had a Greenfield filter in the inferior vena cava to prevent emboli reaching the lungs from the legs following previous thromboembolism, showed very little echogenic material, indicating that the filter acted as an effective block. Inadequate exsanguination of the limb undergoing surgery coupled with stasis and cooling may contribute to fresh thrombus formation. Nevertheless, these 29 patients had echogenic material with clinically adequate exsanguination. Bone cement activation of the coagulation cascade could also form fresh clot. It is likely that the pulmonary circulation is often exposed to embolic material during normal everyday life and that the lungs are able to clear small emboli.

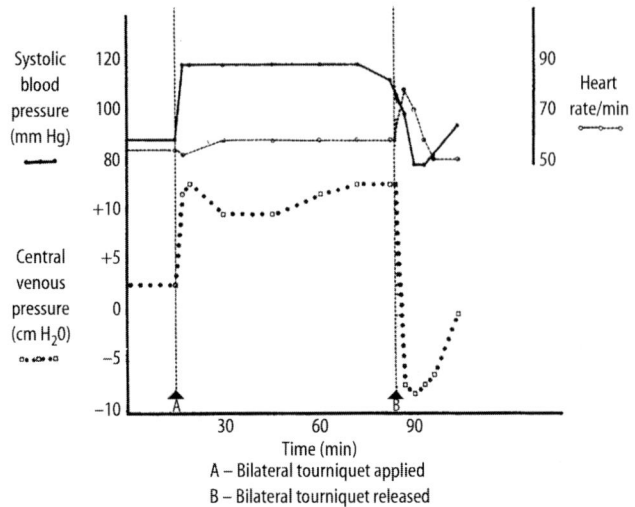

Figure 2.13 Changes in central venous pressure and blood pressure with a tourniquet in place and after release. Reproduced with permission from Bradford, EMW (1968). Haemodynamic changes associated with the application of lower limb tourniquets. *Anaesthesia* 24: 190–197.

2.8 Limb Blood Flow in the Presence of a Tourniquet

The blood supply to the limbs of rhesus monkeys was studied with 50-μ diameter microspheres labelled with ^{51}Cr and by the washout of ^{22}Na injected into the tissues. One limb, upper or lower, was exsanguinated and the circulation was occluded with a pneumatic tourniquet. The opposite limb was used as a control. The blood to the occluded limb was found to be less than 1% of the flow to the control limb. The venous return was less than 0.2% of that of the control limb. It was concluded that a limb with a tourniquet in place is virtually isolated from the circulation and the amount of blood reaching the tissues probably via the intramedullary circulation is likely to be of no significance to relieve the ischaemia.[52] Added support for the isolation of the limb from normal blood flow is provided by the work of Santavirta and colleagues, who studied tissue oxygen levels in rabbits.[53] The tourniquet was in place for 60, 80 or 120 minutes. The baseline PO_2 in the tibialis anterior muscle was 22.6 ± 0.6 mm Hg. While the tourniquet was in place, the oxygen tension dropped to minimal values between 9.2 ± 0.5 and 10.7 ± 0.6 mm Hg in the three groups rendered ischaemic for 60, 80 and 120 minutes, but the tissue microclimate never reached fully anoxic conditions. This minimal value was reached in 19–26 minutes and then remained constant during the remainder of the time that the tourniquet was in place, but it never reached zero. The decline of PO_2 and recovery after release of the tourniquet was independent of tourniquet time. Continuous oxygen during the experiment had no influence on the PO_2.

2.9 Hyperaemia and Swelling of a Limb After Release of a Tourniquet

Using monkeys, a quantitative study was carried out to measure the effect of a tourniquet on the lower limb on peak flow, the amount of swelling, and the time for recovery. The disappearance of acute swelling is related to the period of ischaemia. As the duration of the tourniquet increased, no significant change in peak flow was demonstrated. The swelling that results from a tourniquet for one hour is overcome rapidly, but the effects are much more obvious for tourniquet times of two and three hours. When attempting to obtain haemostasis after release of a tourniquet, surgeons should remember that for a one-hour period of ischaemia, the hyperaemia falls to one-half in about five minutes, but that it takes 12 and 25 minutes, respectively, for this to take place after two and three hours of tourniquet use.[54] These times are of relevance to breathing periods. The onset of hyperaemia is related to the changes brought about by the effects of free oxygen radicals (see Chapter 3).

2.10 Haematological Effects

At the end of orthopaedic operations, there is a pronounced increase in fibrinolytic activity in the blood from the systemic circulation, as well as from the operated limb, whereas there is only a small systemic increase after surgery on the leg without a tourniquet. The vasa vasorum are probably the main source of plasminogen activator in the vasculature and may be stimulated to respond maximally by complete ischaemia; the increase in fibrinolytic activity does not appear to be related to the duration of the application of a tourniquet.[55] However, there is no difference in the incidence of deep vein thrombosis in surgery on the lower limbs with and without a tourniquet.[56] The increase in fibrinolytic activity is short-lived; it is maximal at 15 minutes and returns to preoperative levels within 30 minutes of the release of the tourniquet. It then falls below the preoperative levels, where it remains for at least 48 hours. The tourniquet appears to alter the timing of a short period of increased fibrinolytic activity without altering the overall pattern. It is unlikely that this would alter the incidence of deep vein thrombosis, but it may affect the degree of bleeding after release of the tourniquet.[57]

2.11 Temperature Changes

An increased core body temperature occurs during the application of arterial tourniquets, probably because of reduced metabolic heat transfer from the central to the peripheral compartments and from decreased heat loss from distal skin. When the tourniquet is released, there is a transient decrease in core temperature as a result of redistribution of body heat from the return of hypothermic venous blood flow from the tourniquet limb into the systemic circulation.[58] A marked rise in temperature may cause the anaesthetist concern about the possibility of malignant hyperthermia. An association between the use of tourniquets for limb surgery and a progressive increase in body temperature of greater than one degree with bilateral tourniquets has been reported in children.[59]

With a tourniquet in place, the limb cools gradually; during the course of an operation, the temperature may drop by 3–4 °C. Part of the cooling is counterbalanced by the effects of the lights and drapes in the operation theatre. There may be obvious drying out of the issues exposed, which should always be kept moist with Hartman's solution or normal saline.

2.12 Tourniquet Pain

When a tourniquet is applied to the arms of volunteers, they experience a vague, dull pain in the limb, which is associated with an increase in blood pressure. The average pain tolerance is 31 minutes, increasing to 45 minutes with sedation. Prolonged tourniquet inflation during general anaesthesia causes an increase in heart rate and blood pressure, which commonly leads the anaesthetist to increase the depth of anaesthesia. A cutaneous neural mechanism is thought to be responsible for the tourniquet pain, and the rise in blood pressure follows a humoral response to the pain. Tourniquet pain and the associated hypertension can also complicate spinal or epidural anaesthesia despite adequate sensory anaesthesia of the dermatome underlying the tourniquet.

Tourniquet pain is thought to be transmitted by unmyelinated, slow-conducting C-fibres, which are normally inhibited by fast pain impulses conducted by myelinated A-delta-fibres. Mechanical compression causes loss of conduction due to ischaemia. Large A-delta nerve fibres are blocked, leaving C-fibres still functioning.[16]

Summary

The effect of a tourniquet on the tissues beneath and distal to it have been described. Nerves are vulnerable to high pressures, and muscle is vulnerable to prolonged ischaemia. Based on a study of the ultrastructure of muscle and biochemical changes in the limb subjected to ischaemia in relation to their return to normal, three hours is the upper limit of safety for a tourniquet to be kept in place.

References

1 American Heart Association (1967). Report of a subcommittee of the postgraduate education committee: recommendations for human blood pressure determination by sphygmomanometers. *Circulation* **XXXVI**; 980–988.

2 Pedowitz, RA, Gershuni, DH, Botte, MJ, et al. (1993). The use of lower tourniquet inflation pressures in extremity surgery facilitated by curved and wide tourniquets and an integrated cuff inflation system. *Clinical Orthopaedics and Related Research* **287**: 237–243.

3 Klenerman, L, Hulands, G (1979). Tourniquet pressures for the lower limb. *Journal of Bone and Joint Surgery* **61B**: 124.

4 Lieberman, JR, Staheli, LT, Dales, MC (1997). Tourniquet pressures on paediatric patients: a clinical study. *Orthopaedics* **20**: 1143–1147.

5 Shaw, JA, Murray, DG (1982). The relationship between tourniquet pressure and underlying soft tissue pressure in the thigh. *Journal of Bone and Joint Surgery* **64A**: 1148–1151.

6 Neimkin, RJ, Smith, RJ (1983). Double tourniquet with linked mercury manometers for hand surgery. *Journal of Hand Surgery* **8A**: 938–941.

7 Graham, B, Breault, MJ, McEwen, JA, McGraw, RW (1993). Occlusion of arterial flow in the extremities at subsystolic pressure through the use of wide cuffs. *Clinical Orthopaedics and Related Research* **286**: 257–260.

8 Rydevik, BJ, Lundborg, G, Olmarker, K, Myers RR (2001). Biomechanics of peripheral nerves and spinal nerve roots. In Nordin, M, Frankel, VH, eds. *Basic Biomechanics of the Musculoskeletal System*, 3rd edn. Philadelphia: Lippincott, Williams & Wilkins.

9 Lundborg, G (1988). *Nerve Injury and Repair*. Edinburgh: Churchill Livingstone, p. 83.

10 Yousif, NJ, Grunert, BK, Forte, RA, et al. (1993). A comparison of upper and forearm tourniquet tolerance. *Journal of Hand Surgery* **18B**: 639–641.

11 Hutchinson, DT, McClinton, MA (1993). Upper extremity tourniquet tolerance. *Journal of Hand Surgery* **18A**: 206–210.

12 Odensson, A, Finsen, V (2002). The position of the tourniquet on the upper limb. *Journal of Bone and Joint Surgery* **84B**: 202–204.

13 Michelson, JD, Perry, M (1996). Clinical safety and efficiency of calf tourniquets. *Foot and Ankle International* **17**: 573–575.

14 Lichtenfeld, NS (1992). The pneumatic tourniquet with ankle block anaesthesia for foot surgery. *Foot and Ankle International* **13**: 344–349.

15 Finsen, V, Kasseth, A (1997). Tourniquets in forefoot surgery. Less pain when placed at the ankle. *Journal of Bone and Joint Surgery* **79B**: 99–101.

16 Kam, PCA, Kanaugh, R, Yoong, FFY (2001). The arterial tourniquet: pathophysiological consequences and anaesthetic implications. *Anaesthesia* **56**: 534–545.

17 Bruner, JW (1951). Safety factors in the use of the pneumatic tourniquet for haemostasis in surgery of the hand. *Journal of Bone and Joint Surgery* **33A**: 221–224.

18 Boyes, JH (1964). *Bunnell's Surgery of the Hand*. Philadelphia: J.B. Lippincott and Co., p. 133.

19 Parkes, A (1973). Ischaemic effects of external and internal pressure of the upper limb. *The Hand* **5**: 105–112.

20 Harman, JW, Gwian, RP (1949). The recovery of skeletal muscle fibres from acute ischaemia by histologic and chemical methods. *American Journal of Pathology* **24**: 741–745.

21 Dahlback, LO (1970). Effects of temporary tourniquet ischaemia on striated muscle fibres and motor end-plates. Morphological and histological studies in the rabbit and electromyographical studies in man. *Scandinavian Journal of Plastic and Reconstructive Surgery* Suppl 7.

22 Moore, DH, Ruska, H, Copenhaver, WN (1956). Electromicroscopic and histochemical observations of muscle degeneration after tourniquet. *Journal of Biophysical and Biochemical Cytology* **2**: 755–764.

23 Tountas, CP, Bergman, RA (1977). Tourniquet ischaemia: ultrastructural and histochemical observations of ischaemic human muscle and of monkey muscle and nerve. *Journal of Hand Surgery* **2**: 31–37.

24 Strock, PE, Majino, G (1969). Microvascular changes in acutely ischaemic rat muscle. *Surgery, Gynaecology and Obstetrics* **129**: 1213–1224.

25 Barnard, RJ, Edgerton, VR, Furukaws, T, Peter, JB (1971). Histochemical, biochemical and contractile properties of red, white and intermediate fibres. *American Journal of Physiology* **220**: 410–414.

26 Patterson, S, Klenerman, L (1979). The effect of pneumatic tourniquets on the ultrastructure of skeletal muscle. *Journal of Bone and Joint Surgery* **61B**: 178–183.

27 McAlllister, LP, Munger, BL, Neel, JR (1977). Electron microscopic observations and acid phosphate activity in the ischaemic rat heart. *Journal of Molecular and Cellular Cardiology* **9**: 353–364.

28 Patterson, S, Klenerman, L, Biswas, M, Rhodes, A (1981). The effect of pneumatic tourniquets on skeletal muscle physiology. *Acta Orthopaedica Scandinavica* **52**: 171–175.

29 Mohler, LR, Pedowitz, RA, Lopez, MA, Gershuni, DH (1999). Effects of tourniquet compression on neuromuscular function. *Clinical Orthopaedics and Related Research* **359**: 213–220.

30 Grace, PA (1994). Ischaemic–reperfusion injury. *British Journal of Surgery* **81**: 637–647.

31 Leif, A (1973). Cell swelling a factor in ischaemic tissue injury. *Circulation* **8**: 455–458.

32 Herald, J, Cooper, L, Machart, J (2002). Tourniquet induced restriction of the quadriceps muscle mechanism. *Journal of Bone and Joint Surgery* **84B**: 856–857.

33 Fowler, TJ, Danta, G, Gilliatt, RW (1972). Recovery of nerve conduction after pneumatic tourniquet, observations on the hindlimb of the baboon. *Journal of Neurology, Neurosurgery and Psychiatry* **35**: 638–647.

34 Ochoa, J, Fowler TJ, Gilliatt, RW (1972). Anatomical changes in peripheral nerves compressed by a pneumatic tourniquet. *Journal of Anatomy* **113**: 433–455.

35 Rudge, P, Ochoa, J, Gilliatt, RW (1974). Acute peripheral nerve compression in the baboon. *Journal of Neurological Science* **23**: 403–420.

36 Seddon, H (1943). Three types of nerve injury. *Brain* **66**: 237–288.

37 Gilliatt, RW (1980). Acute compression block. In Sumner, AJ, ed. *The Physiology of Peripheral Nerve Disease.* Philadelphia: W.B. Saunders, pp. 287–315.

38 Dickinson, JC, Bailey, BN (1988). Chemical burns beneath tourniquets. *British Medical Journal* **297**: 1513.

39 Choudhary, S, Koshy, C, Ahmed, J, Evans, J (1998). Friction burns to thigh caused by tourniquet. *British Journal of Plastic Surgery* **51**: 142–143.

40 Parslew, R, Braithwaite, J, Klenerman, L, Friedmann, P (1997). An investigation into the effect of ischaemia and pressure on irritant inflammation. *British Journal of Dermatology* **136**: 734–736.

41 Dery, R, Pelletier, J, Jacques, A, et al. (1965). Metabolic changes induced in the limb during tourniquet ischaemia. *Canadian Anaesthetic Society Journal* **12**: 367–368.

42 Solonen, KA, Takkanen, L, Narvenen, S, Gordin, R (1968). Metabolic changes in the upper limb during tourniquet ischaemia. *Acta Orthopaedica Scandinavica* **39**: 20–22.

43 Stock, W, Bohn, HJ, Isselhard, W (1971). Metabolic changes in rat skeletal muscle after acute arterial occlusion. *Vascular Surgery* **5**: 249–255.

44 Wilgis, EFS (1971). Observations on the effects of tourniquet ischaemia. *Journal of Bone and Joint Surgery* **53A**: 1343–1346.

45 Modig, J, Kolstad, K, Wigren, A (1978). Systemic reactions to tourniquet ischaemia. *Acta Anaesthesiologica Scandinavica* **22**: 609–614.

46 Klenerman, L, Biswas, M, Hulands, GH, Rhodes, AM (1980). Systemic and local effects of the application of a tourniquet. *Journal of Bone and Joint Surgery* **62B**: 385–388.

47 Bradford, EMW (1968). Haemodynamic changes associated with the application of lower limb tourniquets. *Anaesthesia* **24**: 190–197.

48 Kaufman, RD, Walts, LF (1982). Tourniquet induced hypertension. *British Journal of Anaesthesia* **54**: 333–336.

49 Sparling, RJ, Murray, AW, Choksey, M (1993). Raised intracranial pressure associated with raised hypertension after tourniquet removal. *British Journal of Neurosurgery* **7**: 75–78.

50 Berman, AT, Parmet, JR, Harding, SP, et al. (1998). Emboli observed with the use of transoesophageal echocardiography immediately after tourniquet release during total knee arthroplasty with cement. *Journal of Bone and Joint Surgery* **89A**: 389–396.

51 Parmet, JL, Berman, AT, Horrow, JC, et al. (1993). Thromboembolism coincident with tourniquet deflation during total knee arthroplasty. *Lancet* **341**: 1057–1058.

52 Klenerman, L, Crawley, J (1977). Limb blood flow in the presence of a tourniquet. *Acta Orthopaedica Scandinavica* **48**: 291–295.

53 Santavirta, J, Hockerstedt, K, Niinikoski, J (1978). Effect of pneumatic tourniquet on muscle oxygen tension. *Acta Orthopaedica Scandinavica* **49**: 415–419.

54 Klenerman, L, Crawley, J, Lowe, A (1982). Hyperaemia and swelling of a limb upon release of a tourniquet. Acta Orthopaedica Scandinavica **53**: 209–213.

55 Klenerman, L, Mackie, I, Charabarti, R, et al. (1977). Changes in haemostatic system after application of a tourniquet. *Lancet* **1**: 970–972.

56 Angus, PD, Nakielny, R, Gordrum, DT (1983). The pneumatic tourniquet and deep venous thrombosis. *Journal of Bone and Joint Surgery* **65B**: 336–339.

57 Price, AJ, Jones, NAG, Webb, PJ, et al. (1980). Do tourniquets prevent deep vein thrombosis? *Journal of Bone and Joint Surgery* **62B**: 529.

58 Estebe, JP, Le Naoures, A, Malledant, Y, Ecoffey, C (1996). Use of the pneumatic tourniquet induces changes in central temperature. *British Journal of Anaesthesia* **77**: 786–788.

59 Bloch, EC (1986). Hypothermia resulting from tourniquet application in children. *Annals of the Royal College of Surgeons of England* **69**: 193–194.

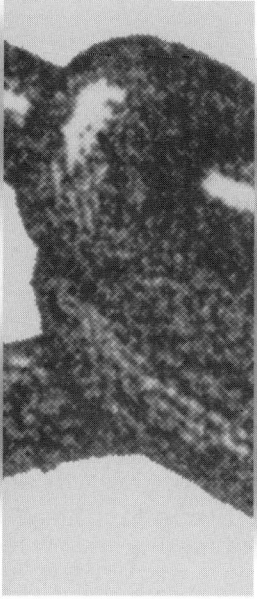

Chapter 3
Ischaemia–Reperfusion Syndrome

BEFORE THE RECOGNITION of reperfusion injury, most studies attributed damage to ischaemia alone and linked reperfusion to the beginning of repair processes and the start of the return to normality. Knowledge of reperfusion injury has shifted the emphasis, perhaps too much, such that some authors have suggested that "ischaemic injury" is a misnomer and that all if not most damage occurs from reperfusion.[1] Probably the correct view is that cell damage following ischaemia is biphasic, with injury being initiated during ischaemia and exacerbated during reperfusion.[2]

Ischaemic injury has been characterised well: the cell is deprived of the energy needed to maintain ionic gradients and homeostasis, and failure of enzyme systems sometimes leads to cell death. Reperfusion injury is mediated by the interaction of free radicals, endothelial factors and neutrophils. While several free-radical species are produced, the most reactive is the hydroxyl radical, which is capable of damaging proteins, DNA and lipids. Lipid peroxidation disrupts cell membranes, which are composed of polyunsaturated fatty acids and phospholipids. The endothelium is a dynamic system that produces several agents that regulate the local environment and may induce neutrophil chemotaxis, adherence and migration. Neutrophils play an important role in systemic injury and cause local tissue destruction by release of proteins and free radicals. The tourniquet as used for orthopaedic surgery provides an excellent example of ischaemia and reperfusion.

3.1 Metabolic Changes

Oxygen as a basic fuel is crucial to all function. Aerobic metabolism replenishes the high-energy phosphate bonds required for cell function. Lack of oxygen results in anaerobic metabolism and an increased concentration of lactic acid. The depletion of cellular stores of energy, especially of adenosine 5′ triphosphate (ATP), results in failure of cellular homeostasis, characterised by loss of ion gradients across the cell membranes.[1] Plasma-membrane changes lead to a loss of sodium and calcium ion imbalance. Sodium ions move into the cell, drawing with them a volume of water to maintain osmotic equilibrium with the surrounding interstitial space. Potassium ions escape from the cell into the interstitium. There is also calcium leakage into the cell, which leads to mitochondrial membrane dysfunction.

3.2 Reperfusion

Restoration of the blood flow has two beneficial consequences for ischaemic tissue: the energy supply is restored and toxic metabolites are removed. The return of toxic

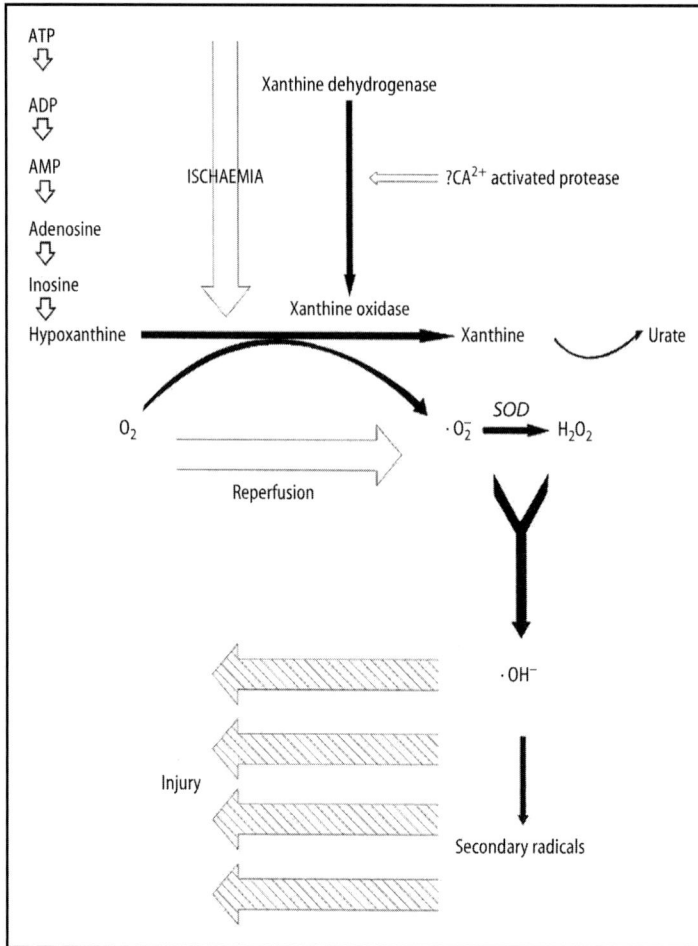

Figure 3.1 Generation of free radicals at reperfusion. Reproduced with permission of Elsevier Science from Bulkley, GB (1994). Reactive oxygen metabolites and reperfusion injury. *Lancet* 334: 934–936.

metabolites to the systemic circulation may have serious metabolic consequences, and reperfusion may also induce further local tissue injury. Free oxygen radicals have been identified as the cause of injury when reperfusion takes place (Figure 3.1).

3.2.1 Oxygen Free Radicals

A free radical is an unstable molecule containing one or more unpaired electrons.[3] In chemical formulae, a superscript dot represents a free radical. Although normally produced in small quantities in a number of sites, including membrane-bound oxidases, phagocytic cells and the electron transport systems of mitochondria, free radicals are rapidly scavenged by various antioxidants that are present locally. Free radicals have extremely high reactivity and exist for a very short period. They are also frequently involved in reactions that can be self-perpetuating, and they set the stage for the generation of multiple chain reactions, e.g. several oxygen free radicals may be produced by reduction or excitation of molecular oxygen. The unpaired superoxide radical ($\cdot O_2$) is formed by the addition of one electron to a molecule of oxygen. Superoxide can inactivate specific enzymes and is the precursor of hydrogen peroxide and the highly reactive hydroxyl radical. The superoxide dismutases (SODs) found in mitochondria and the cytoplasm convert superoxide to hydrogen peroxide and oxygen:

$$2 \cdot O_2 + 2H^+ \rightarrow H_2O_2 + O_2$$

The hydrogen peroxide generated is destroyed by catalase:

$$2 H_2O_2 \rightarrow 2 H_2O + O_2$$

If it is not removed completely, the hydrogen peroxide may react with the superoxide in the presence of iron to form the hydroxyl free radical:

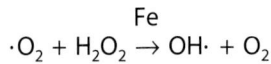

$$\overset{\text{Fe}}{\cdot O_2 + H_2O_2 \rightarrow OH\cdot + O_2}$$

The hydroxyl radical is the most reactive of the free oxygen radicals in biological systems and is probably responsible for most of the cellular damage that occurs from free radicals.[4] Hydrogen peroxide generated through the dismutation of superoxide reacts with ferrous ions to produce a family of related free radicals. This second reaction of hydrogen peroxide and ferrous ions is called the Haber–Weiss reaction and is noted for the generation of the highly cytotoxic hydroxyl ($\cdot OH$) radical. The enzyme xanthine oxidase is potentially a major source of free radicals in reperfused ischaemic tissue. Free radicals are capable of damaging all biomolecules and may therefore lead to many of the features of reperfusion injury. Their inherent high reactivity means that they react close to the site of generation and hence may be difficult to scavenge in the tissues.

3.2.2 Neutrophil Polymorphonuclear Leucocytes (Neutrophils)

Local and systemic damage is associated with neutrophil accumulation in the microvasculature. Neutrophil–endothelial cell reactions are a prerequisite for microvascular injury. Activated neutrophils adhere to and migrate across the endothelium and cause local destruction by releasing free radicals, proteolytic enzymes and peroxidases.

3.2.3 Defence Mechanisms

Several endogenous mechanisms exist to inhibit ischaemic reperfusion injury. In addition, some drugs have been found to be effective. Free-radical scavengers interact with reactive oxygen species to render them harmless. Catalase is a naturally occurring metalloproteinase that catalyses the formation of water and oxygen from hydrogen peroxide and acts with superoxide dismutase in vivo. Mannitol has been used clinically for its hydroxyl-radical-scavenging effects for many years.[5]

3.2.4 Swelling After Ischaemia

Swelling is an invariable consequence of tourniquet use. It contributes to post-operative pain. The increase in vascular permeability is linked to the inflammatory response started by free-radical action on endothelial cells. Water moves into the cell, accompanying the fluxes of sodium and calcium ions. There is an increased interstitial pressure within the rigid fascial compartments of the upper and lower limbs, which contributes to the collapse of the microvasculature and impairment of the blood supply. In a study in which heparin was administered before application of the tourniquet, there was less oedema after the tourniquet was released, suggesting that some intravascular thrombosis is probably involved in the production of swelling.[6]

3.3 Modifying Ischaemia–Reperfusion

3.3.1 Pharmacological Modification

Pharmacological modification of ischaemia-reperfusion injury has been directed at reducing the production and efforts of superoxide and secondary radicals at several levels (Figure 3.2). Generation of superoxide has been modified using allopurinol, a xanthine oxidase inhibitor,[7] whereas secondary production of the more cytotoxic hydroxyl radical is influenced by desferrioxamine, an iron chelator.[8] The complexity of reperfusion injury and tissue differences in free-radical production accounts for the lag in success in clinical compared with animal studies.

Pharmacological intervention to reduce post-ischaemic injury has been directed at other important mechanisms of damage. Intracellular accumulation of calcium, either from extracellular fluid or the sarcoplasmic reticulum, is implicated in this injury. Calcium-release modulators such as dantrolene have been shown to provide partial protection against reperfusion injury.[9] The effect of four hours of ischaemia followed by reperfusion for one hour was studied in anaesthetised rabbits. Muscles of the limb to which the tourniquets had been applied showed considerable ultrastructural damage, although the distribution of damage between muscles was not uniform (in descending order of damage: anterior tibial, soleus, quadriceps).

Damage to the muscle was associated with a significant increase in the concentration of some indicators of free-radical-mediated processes (thiobarbituric acid reactive substances and diene conjugates), although others (glutathione and protein sulphydryl groups) were unchanged. Reperfused muscles also showed considerable increase in their calcium and sodium contents.

Treatment with dantrolene sodium (4 mg/h) throughout the periods of ischaemia and reperfusion was found to preserve the ultrastructural appearance of the quadriceps, soleus and anterior tibial muscles. No effect of dantrolene sodium on indicators of free radical activity or muscle calcium contents was seen.

In a further investigation, the same group examined the potential protective effect of pretreatment with corticosteroids or antioxidants (ascorbic acid or allopurinol) in

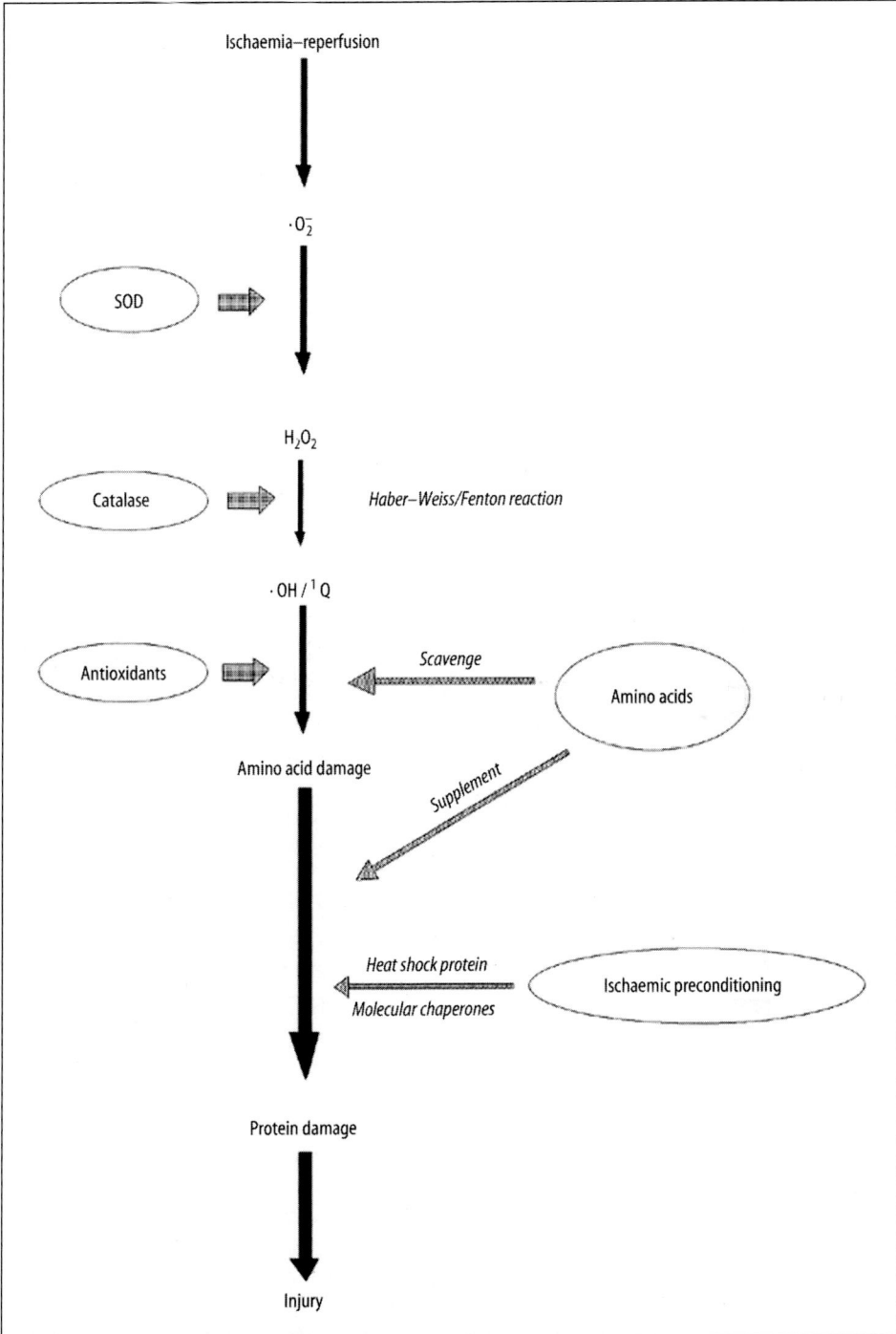

Figure 3.2 Protective strategies in reducing ischaemia–reperfusion injury. Reproduced with permission from Kukreja, RC, Hess, ML (1992). The oxygen free radical system: from equations through membrane–protein interactions to cardiovascular injury and protection. *Cardiovascular Research* 26: 641–645.

rabbits with damage to skeletal muscle after reperfusion for one hour, following four hours of ischaemia with pneumatic tourniquets on a hind limb.[10] There was a considerable amount of ultrastructural damage to the anterior tibial muscles accompanied by a rise in circulating creatine kinase activity.

Pretreatment of animals with depot methylprednisolone by a single 8-mg intramuscular injection led to preservation of the structure of tibialis anterior on both light and electron microscopy. High-dose, continuous intravenous infusion with ascorbic acid (80 mg/h) throughout the period of ischaemia and reperfusion also preserved the structure of the muscle. Allopurinol in various doses had no effect.

These findings are fully compatible with a mechanism of ischaemia–reperfusion-induced injury, involving generation of oxygen radicals and neutrophil sequestration and activation. The findings indicate that damage to human skeletal muscle caused by prolonged use of a tourniquet is likely to be reduced by simple pharmacological intervention.

3.3.2 Physical Modification

The practice of using breathing periods represents an attempt to reduce ischaemic injury. This involves releasing the tourniquet after a set period of ischaemia to allow reperfusion, with the aim of returning tissue to its pre-ischaemic state, before subjecting the limb to a further period of ischaemia. Several studies have defined the appropriate breathing periods for the time ischaemia is required.

Newman, on the basis of studies in rats with nuclear magnetic resonance (NMR) spectroscopy, suggested that the biochemical determinant of the speed of recovery after the release of the tourniquet was the level of ATP.[10] Rapid recovery always occurred in the presence of ATP but not in its absence. He found that hourly ten-minute breather periods prevented the depletion of ATP, and hence during three hours of ischaemia the metabolic demands for chemical energy were met. If the interval was only five minutes, this did not prevent ATP depletion and in addition to causing a deterioration of tissue pH did not shorten the recovery time. Pedowitz, using technetium uptake, found in a rabbit model that with a tourniquet time of four hours, skeletal muscle injury beneath the cuff was reduced significantly by hourly ten-minute reperfusion intervals.[11] He noted that a ten-minute reperfusion period after a two-hour tourniquet tended to exacerbate muscle injury. Reperfusion intervals could prolong the duration of anaesthesia, increase blood loss, or produce haemorrhagic staining and oedema.[12] Nevertheless, Sapega and colleagues recommended on the basis of studies on dogs that ischaemic injury to muscle can be minimised by limiting the initial period of tourniquet time to 1.5 hours.[13] Release of the tourniquet for five minutes permitted a further period of 1.5 hours. With knowledge of the ischaemia–reperfusion syndrome, the use of breathing periods is not logical, as reperfusion is now recognised as a major cause of damage to limbs after ischaemia. Further damage by free-radical-mediated mechanisms is likely even after the biochemistry of the venous blood returns to normal equilibrium. Work in animals has suggested that allowing reperfusion may actually increase the amount of damage to the ischaemic limb in certain structures.[14]

3.3.3 Hypothermia

The beneficial effects of hypothermia on the survival of ischaemic tissue have been shown in various studies.[6] The underlying basis for protection is thought to be a reduction in the rate of cellular metabolism and, as such, may influence both ischaemia and reperfusion mechanisms of injury. A successful, prospective, randomised study was carried out on the hind limbs of pigs.[15] Significant slowing of metabolism was shown in hypothermic ischaemic limbs through measurement of high levels of muscle glycogen and phosphofructose. The difference was detectable several days after cooling and use of a tourniquet. In addition, the rate of return to normal levels of serum lactate, serum potassium and pH in hypothermic limbs suggested less tissue damage and a lower oxygen debt.

Nayagam carried out a randomised, prospective trial of the role of hypothermia in a series of 19 patients undergoing knee replacements, divided into cooled and control groups.[16] The effect of tourniquet ischaemia on muscle was considered separately from reperfusion injury. The effect of preoperative limb cooling was assessed using clinical variables as well as biochemical assays of tissue samples. The Richard King Limb Cooler (SI Industries, Croydon, UK) is simple and easy to apply and allows precise control of temperature. The target was 15 °C below skin temperature at the start or the lowest cooling that was reached that could be tolerated. Muscle biopsies from vastus medialis each amounting to 50–60 mg were taken at the start of the operation, just before release of the tourniquet and just before closure of the skin. Times were noted when the biopsies were taken, so the period of ischaemia and reperfusion for each sample was known. All samples were wrapped in foil and stored immediately in liquid nitrogen. The assays showed highly significant rises in intramuscular sodium and calcium during the ischaemic period. In the control group, the influx of sodium was proportional to tourniquet time. Potassium and magnesium levels remained unchanged during this period. On reperfusion, there was a highly significant decrease in potassium in the control group. The cooled group showed a similar trend, but the values were not statistically significant. Sodium and calcium levels did not change significantly in either group in this phase.

These results suggest that significant injury occurs during ischaemia, as shown by the movement of calcium and sodium ions. The loss of ATP alters the function of cation pumps within the plasma membrane. The influence of preoperative cooling is moderate; sodium influx, which was proportional to tourniquet time in the control group, appears to lose the relationship on cooling. The effect of preoperative cooling on reperfusion is clear as there is a significant reduction in the loss of magnesium and potassium. The manner by which this is brought about remains unclear, since the level of thiobarbituric acid reacting substances (TBARS) produced from lipid peroxidation of plasma membranes was the same in both groups. Preoperative cooling had no effect on TBARS. This may be due to the relatively small impact on metabolism due to the 5°C difference in temperature on the cooled group, since breakdown of ATP to hypoxanthine may not have been reduced.

Patients who had preoperative cooling lost a significantly smaller volume of blood (P 0.05). This difference may have been a reflection of persistent vasoconstriction in the cooled group after the release of the tourniquet. This was seen even 20 minutes after release of the tourniquet. The difference in blood loss is approximately one unit of blood and, at these volumes, may amount to a decision not to transfuse.

With regard to postoperative pain, there was a significant difference in visual analogue scores measured eight and 24 hours postoperatively. A placebo effect could not be excluded.

3.3.4 Ischaemic Preconditioning of Skeletal Muscle

Ischaemic preconditioning is a process by which exposure of a tissue to a short period of (non-damaging) ischaemic stress leads to resistance to the deleterious effects of a subsequent prolonged ischaemic stress. It has been described extensively in the heart, but few studies have examined the possibility that it can occur in skeletal muscle. A rat model of unilateral limb ischaemia has been used to examine this possibility. Exposure of the hind limb to a five-minute period of ischaemia and a five-minute period of reperfusion significantly protected the tibialis anterior muscle against the structural damage induced by a subsequent period of four hours of limb ischaemia and one hour of reperfusion.[17, 18] This protection was evident on examination of muscle by both light and electron microscopy. Longer or shorter times of prior ischaemia had no effect. Prior exposure of the hind limb to five minutes of ischaemia and five minutes of reperfusion did not prevent the fall in ATP in the tibialis anterior muscle that occurred following a subsequent four-hour period of ischaemia and one hour of reperfusion. Similarly, no effect of the programme of preconditioning on the elevated muscle myeloperoxidase (indicative of a raised neutrophil content) or abnormal muscle cation contents was seen. Reperfused ischaemic muscle was found to have an increased content of heat shock protein (HSP) 72. The preconditioning protocol did not increase the content of this or other HSPs further, which indicates that it was not acting by increasing the protection of these cytoprotective proteins. The protective effects of preconditioning appear to be reproduced by infusion of adenosine to animals immediately before the four-hour period of ischaemia. This indicates a potential mechanism by which skeletal muscle may be preconditioned to maintain structural viability, as adenosine inhibits free-radical production from activated neutrophils via a receptor-mediated mechanism.[19]

The use of breathing periods can now be abandoned and replaced by perioperative pharmacological protection, such as intravenous adenosine before release of the tourniquet, but proof of this is still required in clinical practice.

Summary

The role of free oxygen radicals has been described in relation to the ischaemia–reperfusion syndrome, which has given a new perspective on the changes after the application and release of a tourniquet. Protection by physical and pharmacological means is possible. Breathing periods are no longer applicable.

References

1 McCord, JM (1985). Oxygen-derived free radicals in postischaemic tissue injury. *New England Journal of Medicine* **312**: 156–163.

2 Grace, PA (1994). Ischaemia–reperfusion injury. *British Journal of Surgery* **81**: 637–647.

3 Dormandy, TL (1989). Free radical pathology and medicine. A review. *Journal of the Royal College of Physicians of London* **23**: 221–227.

4 Haber, J, Weiss, J (1934). The catalytic decomposition of hydrogen peroxide by iron salts. *Proceedings of the Royal Society. Series A* **147**; 332–351.

5 Magovem, GJ, Bolling, SF, Casale, AS, et al. (1984). The mechanism of mannitol in reducing ischaemic injury: hyperosmolarity or hydroxyl scavenger. *Circulation* **10** (suppl 1): 191–195.

6 Oredsson, S, Plate, G, Quarfordt, P (1991). Allopurinol – a free radical scavenger – reduces reperfusion injury in skeletal muscle. *European Journal of Vascular Surgery* **5**: 47–52.

7 Ambrosio, G, Zweier, JL, Jacobus, WE, et al. (1987). Improvement of postischaemic myocardial function and metabolism induced by administration of deferoxamine at the time of reflow: the role of iron in the pathogenesis of reperfusion injury. *Circulation* **76**: 907–915.

8 Klenerman, L, Lowe, N, Miller, I, et al. (1995). Dantrolene sodium protects against experimental ischaemia. *Acta Orthopaedica Scandinavica* **66**: 352–358.

9 Bushell, A, Klenerman, L, Davies, H, et al. (1996). Ischaemia–reperfusion-induced muscle damage. Protective effect of corticosteroids and anti-oxidants in rabbits. *Acta Orthopaedica Scandinavica* **66**: 393–398.

10 Newman, RJ (1984). Metabolic effects of tourniquets ischaemia studied by nuclear magnetic resonance spectroscopy. *Journal of Bone and Joint Surgery* **66B**: 434–440.

11 Pedowitz, AR, Gershuni, DH, Friden, J, et al. (1992). Effects of reperfusion intervals on skeletal muscle injury beneath and distal to a pneumatic tourniquet. *Journal of Hand Surgery* **17A**: 245–255.

12 Concannon, MJ, Kester, CG, Welsh, CF, Puckett, CL (1992). Patterns of free radical production after tourniquet ischaemia: implications for the hand surgeon. *Plastic and Reconstructive Surgery* **89**: 846–851.

13 Sapega, AA, Heppenstall, RB, Chanc, B, et al. (1985). Optimising tourniquet application and release times in extremity surgery. *Journal of Bone and Joint Surgery* **67A**; 303–314.

14 Paletta, FX, Shehadi, SI, Mudd, JG, Cooper, T. Hypothermia and tourniquet ischaemia (1962). *Plastic and Reconstructive Surgery* **29**: 531–538.

15 Irving, G, Noakes, TD (1985). The protective role of local hypothermia in tourniquet induced ischaemia of muscle. *Journal of Bone and Joint Surgery* **67B**: 297–301.

16 Nayagam, S (1995). Limb cooling in knee replacement surgery: modulating ischaemia–reperfusion injury. Master of Orthopaedic Surgery thesis. Liverpool: University of Liverpool.

17 Bushell, AJ, Klenerman, L, Taylor, S, et al. (2002). Ischaemic preconditioning of skeletal muscle. 1. Protection against the structural changes induced by ischaemia/reperfusion injury. *Journal of Bone and Joint Surgery* **84B**: 1184–1187.

18 Bushell, A, Klenerman, L, Davies, H, et al (2002). Ischaemic preconditioning of skeletal muscle. 2. Investigation of the mechanisms involved. *Journal of Bone and Joint Surgery* **84B**: 1189–1193.

19 Cronstein, BN, Rosenstein, ED, Kramer, SB, et al. (1985). Adenosine: a physiological modulator of superoxide anion generation by human neutrophils. *Journal of Immunology* **135**: 1366–1371.

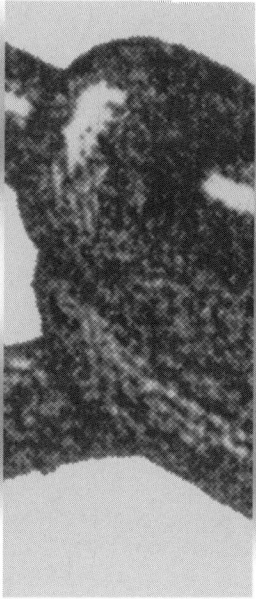

Chapter 4
Exsanguination of the Limb

BEFORE THE TOURNIQUET is inflated, it is essential to empty the limb of as much blood as possible. This prevents unnecessary oozing and helps precise anatomical dissection.

When Lister used a tourniquet in 1879 to help him radically excise tuberculous wrist joints, he was aware of the need for preliminary elevation of the limb.[1] He was fascinated by the mechanism of blanching of the hand when it was elevated to 90 degrees, and he was convinced that this was brought about by the nervous system. He described simple experiments in a volunteer, and he also experimented on an anaesthetised horse. In a lecture to the Harveian Society, Lister described how his attention had been drawn to the problem about 15 years previously. He advocated preliminary elevation for a few minutes before the application of a tourniquet.

Distefano and colleagues, using impedance plethysmography, found that the maximal decrease in volume by elevation alone, with the limb at 45 degrees, occurred after 15–20 seconds, with no noticeable change thereafter.[2] While any changes in impedance theoretically represent changes in intravascular and extravascular compartments, in this study it would reflect only the former. Warren and colleagues, measuring changes of circumference of the limb with mercury in silastic strain gauges, found that the optimal time for elevation was five minutes.[3] For the maximal effect, they suggested that the upper limb should be elevated at 90 degrees; for the lower limb, they suggested 45 degrees of elevation, since further elevation was likely to kink the femoral vein due to the flexion of the hip.

Using a gamma-camera technique and the injection of autologous 99m technetium-labelled erythrocytes, Blond and colleagues showed that there was little change in the reduction of blood volume of the lower limb at 60 degrees with an increase of the duration of elevation.[4, 5] The results after half a minute were 45%, one minute 45%, two minutes 43%, four minutes 44%, six minutes 43%, and ten minutes 44%. This pattern was also seen in the upper limb.

4.1 External Compression

External compression in addition to elevation has been shown to improve the degree of exsanguination However, it is contraindicated in patients who have a suspected infected or malignant lesion. Use of an Esmarch bandage or hand-over-hand manual exsanguination[6] are more effective than elevation alone.

Use of an Esmarch bandage is time-consuming and can damage the skin over a fracture or the atrophic skin of a patient with rheumatoid arthritis (Figure 4.1). It can also detach pre-existing venous thromboses and produce pulmonary emboli.[7–9]

Furthermore, there is no effective control of the pressure with which an Esmarch bandage is applied. Undue stretching as each turn is applied results in increased pressure. The average tension produced on routine application is 125 N; 175 N is near the tensile limit of the bandage.[10] Martin's bandage made of cream-coloured latex rubber is used in a similar manner.

Sterilisation of an Esmarch bandages requires care but is effective if the bandage is rolled loosely with a gauze bandage between the layers and placed in an autoclave.[11]

For knee surgery, the adequacy of exsanguination produced by an Esmarch bandage has been compared with the effect of elevation for two minutes.[12] A blinded, randomised, prospective trial was undertaken in 50 patients having total knee replacement and 50 patients having arthroscopy. The mean blood loss during total knee replacement was significantly greater in the group that was elevated. The haematocrit of samples of arthroscopy drainage was consistently less than 1%, irrespective of the method of exsanguination. None of the operating surgeons reported that they considered that the surgery had been made more difficult by the use of elevation alone. With elevation, the skin and superficial tissues are not cleared of blood as effectively as with an Esmarch bandage. Minimal superficial bleeding did not interfere with the surgical procedure at a deeper level. It was concluded that considering the established risks of Esmarch bandages and the adequacy of the field provided by elevation, the latter method was preferable. In contrast, Strover, in a large personal series, did not use a tourniquet or mention exsanguination for either arthroscopies or total knee replacements.[13]

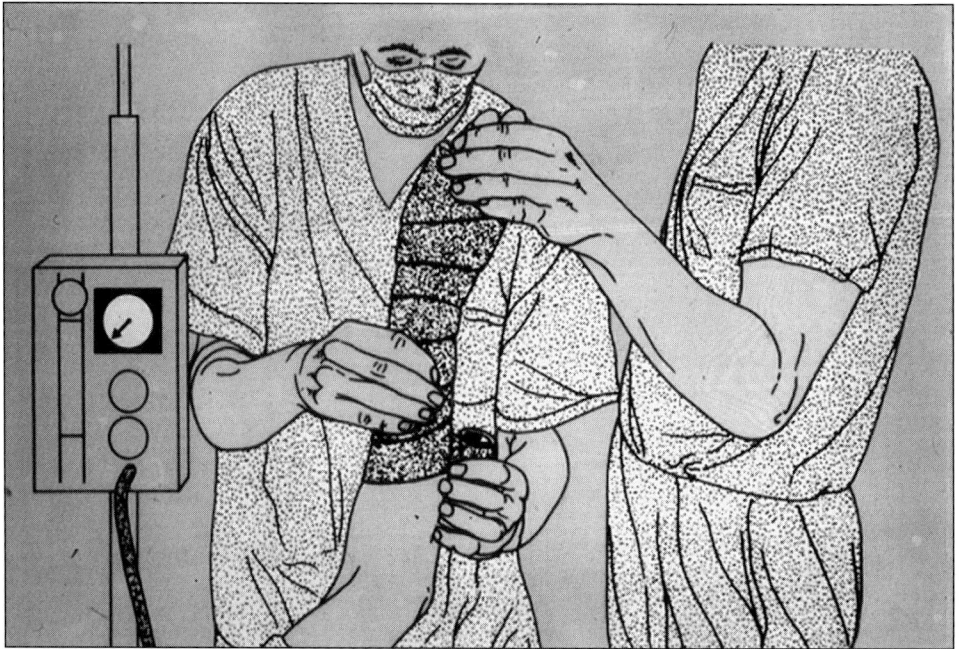

Figure 4.1 Application of an Esmarch bandage. By keeping close to the limb, one can avoid undue tension.

A technique described by Burchell and Stack[14] was later modified in the form of the Northwick Park Hospital Exsanguinator.[15] Use of this apparatus did not require elevation of the limb and thus could be used single-handedly. The apparatus consisted of a plastic cover applied to the limb distal to the tourniquet and inflated to systolic pressure for one minute for exsanguination, before the tourniquet was inflated. The splint was then deflated and removed.

In a similar manner, an arm splint used for the stabilisation of fractures for transport was inflated by compressed air to a pressure of 200 mm Hg. The tourniquet was then inflated. The splint was deflated, unzipped and removed before intravenous regional anaesthesia was given (see Chapter 6).[16]

The need for control of the pressure that is applied has led to the development of appliances such as the Rhys-Davies Exsanguinator.[17] This is an inflated elastic cylinder that is rolled on to the limb (Figure 4.2). As the exsanguinator is applied, the pressure within the sleeve increases. With small limbs, this is not marked and the degree of exsanguination is less. On a very large limb, the maximum pressure generated is

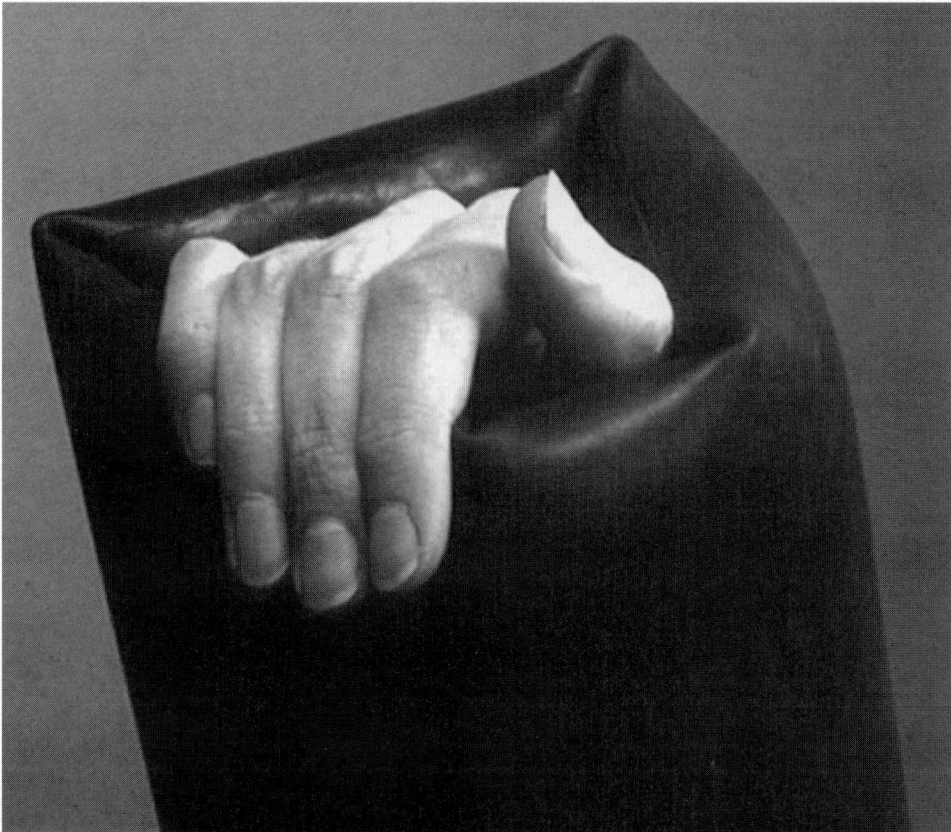

Figure 4.2 Use of the Rhys-Davies Exsanguinator: (a) Preliminary grip.

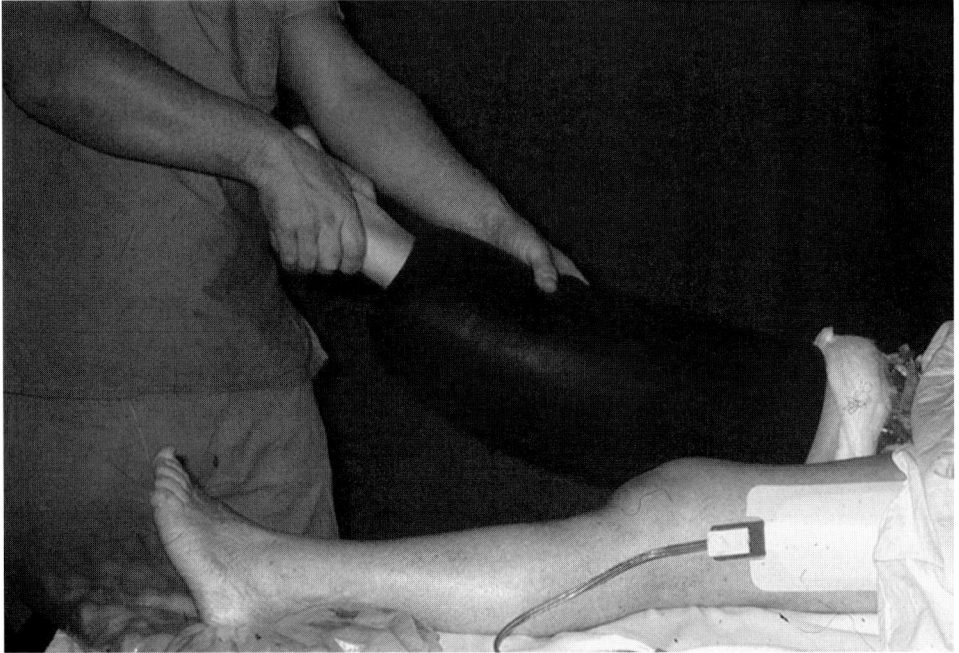

Figure 4.2 (b) Starting on the limb.

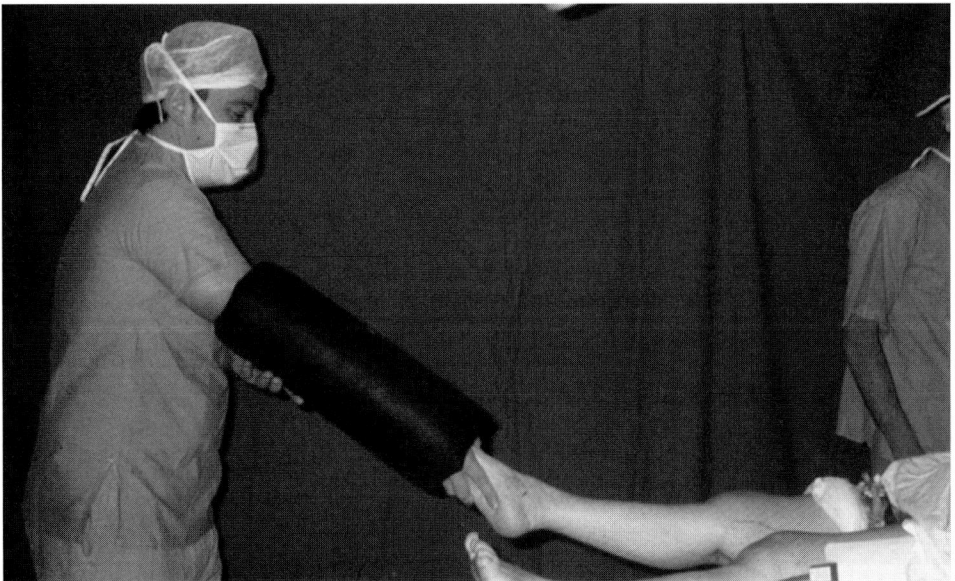

Figure 4.2 (c) Completion.

only about 150 mm Hg, which is distributed uniformly over the whole exposed surface of the limb. The exsanguinator does not produce localised ridges of high pressure or distort superficial tissues. Reinflation and direct measurement of the inflation pressure are done through a valve in the wall of the cylinder, and a sphygmomanometer cuff is rolled up inside it. The exsanguinator requires regular maintenance, and the manufacturer recommends that it be replaced annually.

External methods of exsanguination reduce limb volume by forcing blood from it. Using a water-displacement method, Silver and colleagues showed that a limb would swell immediately by approximately 10% of its original volume after release of a pneumatic tourniquet (Figure 4.3).[18] About half of the swelling is due to the return of the exsanguinated blood to the limb. Further swelling is an effect of reactive hyperaemia, and additional swelling can occur following both haematoma formation due to surgery and the accumulation of oedema from anoxia. Therefore, the postoperative dressing must allow for this inevitable swelling (Figure 4.4). A plaster should never be completely circumferential; instead, it should be split in the midline or applied only as a backslab, or there should be a well-padded dressing.

In summary, the combination of elevation and the use of a Rhys-Davies Exsanguinator is a safe and easy method for daily practice and can be used without fear of complications.

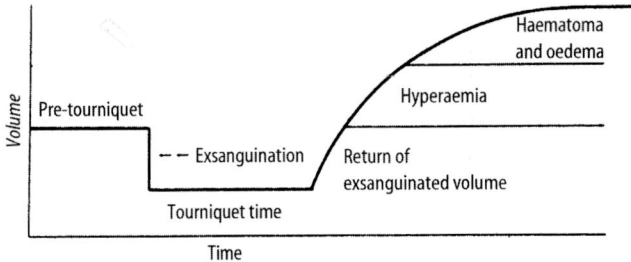

Figure 4.3 To show changes in volume occurring after exsanguination. Reproduced with permission of Lippincott, Williams & Wilkins from Silver, R, de la Garza, J, Koreska, J, Rang, M (1986). Limb swelling after release of tourniquets. *Clinical Orthopaedics* 206: 86–89.

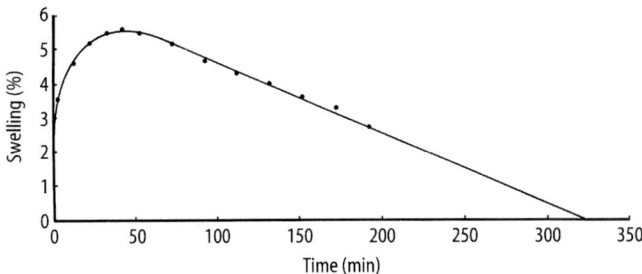

Figure 4.4 Effect on the volume of the limb, as seen in a rabbit's hind limb, following deflation after application of a tourniquet for three hours.

4.2 Sickle Cell Disease

The role of exsanguination and the use of tourniquets are controversial in patients with sickle cell disease. Sickle cell disease is common in the West Indies and West Africa. The erythrocytes assume a crescent-like or sickle shape when deprived of oxygen. Blood that remains in a limb distal to a tourniquet may sickle. Tourniquets induce the three most critical conditions known to produce sickling: circulatory stasis, acidosis and hypoxia. Homozygous patients with erythrocytes containing the abnormal haemoglobin S are at risk, but heterozygous patients who have the sickle cell trait but also normal haemoglobin A are not at risk. Sickle cell trait is the result of inheritance of normal haemoglobin from one parent and haemoglobin S from the other. The small proportion of haemoglobin S is of less clinical significance, although it is not completely innocuous. The erythrocytes contain enough haemoglobin S to sickle in the laboratory preparation. Ludham and Jellis, working in Zambia, pointed out that a bloodless field may shorten the time taken for surgery, make surgery safer, and minimise blood loss, especially if no blood is available for transfusion.[19] Conversely, blood that remains in the limb may sickle, with potentially serious effects. With careful monitoring of systemic pO_2 by pulse oximetry, Ludham and Jellis have not seen any marked lowering after deflation of the tourniquet in patients with sickle cell disease. The benefits afforded by the use of a tourniquet need to be balanced against the dangers, and a decision should be made for each individual operation. Careful exsanguination is the key to safety. This approach accords with the report of Stein and Urbaniak, who found in a series of 21 patients carrying the sickle cell gene and who underwent 29 operations under tourniquet that there was no statistically increased incidence of complications when compared with a control group of black patients without the sickle cell trait and who had similar operations.[20]

References

1 Godlee, RJ (1924). *Lord Lister*, 3rd edn. Oxford: Clarendon Press. p. 632.

2 Distefano, V, Nixon, JE, Stone, RH (1974). Bioelectric impedance plethysmography as an investigative tool in orthopaedic surgery – a comparative study of limb exsanguination techniques. *Clinical Orthopaedics* **99**: 203–206.

3 Warren, PJ, Hardman, PJ, Woolf, VJ (1992). Limb exsanguination. i. The arm: effects of angle of elevation and arterial compression. ii. The leg: effects of angle of elevation. *Annals of the Royal College of Surgeons of England* **74**: 320–322, 323–325.

4 Blond, L, Kirketorp-Moller, K, Sonne-Holm, S, Madsen, JL (2002). Exsanguination of lower limb in healthy male subjects. *Acta Orthopaedica Scandinavica* **73**: 89–92.

5 Blond, L, Madsen, JL (2002). Exsanguination of the upper limb in healthy young volunteers. *Journal of Bone and Joint Surgery* **84B**: 489–491.

6 Colville, J, Small, JO (1986). Exsanguination of the upper limb in hand surgery – comparison of four methods. *The Hand* **11B**: 469–470.

7 Austin, M (1963). The Esmarch bandage and pulmonary embolism. *Journal of Bone and Joint Surgery* **45B**: 384–385.

8 Pollard, BJ, Lovelock, HA, Jones, RM (1983). Fatal pulmonary embolism secondary to limb exsanguination. *Anaesthesiology* **58**: 373–374.

9 Hoffman, A, Wyatt, RWB (1985). Fatal pulmonary embolism following tourniquet inflation. *Journal of Bone and Joint Surgery* **67A**: 633–634.

10 McClaren, AC, Rorabeck, CH (1985). The pressure distribution under tourniquets. *Journal of Bone and Joint Surgery* **67A**: 433–438.

11 O'Hara, JN, Coleman, M, Hutton, RM (1991). A simple and effective method of sterilizing Esmarch bandages. *Journal of Arthroplasty* **6**: 95–96.

12 Marshall, PD, Patel, M, Fairclough, JA (1994). Should Esmarch bandages be used for exsanguination in knee arthroscopy and knee replacement surgery? A prospective trial of Esmarch exsanguination versus simple elevation. *Journal of the Royal College of Surgeons of Edinburgh*; **38**: 189–190.

13 Strover, A (1996). Are tourniquets in total knee replacement and arthroscopy necessary? *The Knee* **3**: 115–119.

14 Burchell, G, Stack, G (1993). Exsanguination of the arm and hand. *The Hand* **5**: 124–126.

15 Klenerman, L (1978). A modified tourniquet: preliminary communication. *Journal of the Royal Society of Medicine* **71**: 121–122.

16 Winnie, AP, Ramamurthy, S (1970). Pneumatic exsanguination for intravenous regional anaesthesia. *Anaesthesiology* **33**: 664–665.

17 Rhys-Davies, NC, Stotter, AT (1985). The Rhys-Davies Exsanguinator. *Annals of the Royal College of Surgeons of England* **67**: 193–195.

18 Silver, R, de la Garza, J, Koreska, J, Rang, M (1986). Limb swelling after release of tourniquets. *Clinical Orthopaedics* **206**: 86–89.

19 Ludham, CA, Jellis, J (2002). Blood disorders and AIDS. In Benson, M, Fixsen, JA, MacNicol, M, Parch, K, eds. *Children's Clinical Orthopaedics and Fractures*, 2nd edn. London: Churchill Livingstone, p. 116.

20 Stein, RE, Urbaniak, J (1980). Use of tourniquet during surgery in patients with sickle cell haemoglobinopathies. *Clinical Orthopaedics* **151**: 231–233.

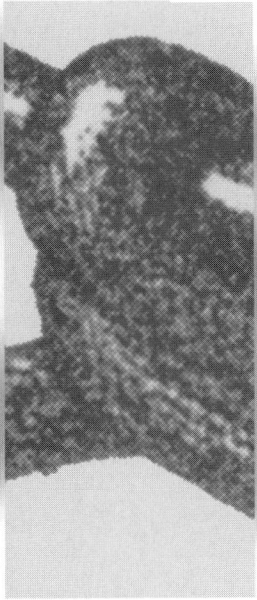

Chapter 5
Complications

A TOURNIQUET CAN damage any of the tissues of a limb. Complications arise because of failure to treat the limb physiologically and should be preventable. In addition, there is an inevitable complication that always follows the use of a tourniquet to some extent: swelling. Swelling is related directly to the duration of ischaemia, and it must be anticipated. Release of the tourniquet and haemostasis before the wound is closed will help to reduce swelling. There should be space available in well-padded postoperative dressings, and the limb should be elevated for the first few hours after operation. The effects of swelling must not be aggravated by constrictive dressings or plaster casts. Complete plasters must never be applied unless they are split immediately. Backslabs are preferred, since these avoid the possibility of compartment syndrome due to external compression.

Complications often have medicolegal implications. The most common problems, in my experience, are nerve lesions, burns following spirit-based antiseptic solutions seeping beneath the cuff, and failure to recognise peripheral vascular disease before the operation, which may lead to delayed wound healing or even amputation.

5.1 Damage to Nerves

Harvey Cushing introduced the use of a pneumatic tourniquet because of the problems of nerve injuries produced by Esmarch bandages and solid rubber tourniquets. Speigel and Lewin[1] claim that the first available reports of tourniquet paralysis are those of Montes, recorded in a Mexican journal, and Putnam, recorded in a report to the Boston Society for Medical Improvement.[2] The largest series of similar cases is that collected by Eckhoff, who described 14 patients.[3] Eckhoff stated: "no effort is too great in the prevention of this condition". He hoped his article would stimulate the routine use of a pneumatic tourniquet. In his series, most lesions recovered within three months.

Middleton and Varian investigated the number of neurological complications after the use of a tourniquet by means of a questionnaire sent to 151 members of the Australian Orthopaedic Association.[4] The incidence of peripheral nerve lesions was one in 5000 for the arm and one in 13 000 for the leg. The arm palsies fell into two main groups: the largest group involved median, ulnar and radial nerves below the tourniquet, while the slightly smaller group comprised isolated radial nerve lesions. The lesions occurred with both Esmarch bandages and pneumatic cuffs. All except one patient made a full recovery; the exception developed a complete radial nerve injury, which persisted. The approximate time for recovery was four to five months, although some palsies were transient and others required up to 12 months to disappear.

In the lower limb, all the nerve lesions reported by Middleton and Varian were produced by Esmarch bandages. Rorabeck and Kennedy have reported five cases of sciatic nerve injury after pneumatic tourniquets.[5] The pressure in all cases was 500 mm Hg. A standard Kidde tourniquet was used. The tourniquet time varied from 45 to 90 minutes. All patients had an obvious neurological defect immediately after their operation. There was a complete absence of function in both the lateral and medial popliteal divisions in one patient, and a partial foot drop was seen in four patients. Guanche reported a single case of posterior tibial nerve palsy following the use of a pneumatic tourniquet.[6] This was in contrast to Rorabeck and Kennedy, who found the lateral popliteal to be affected most commonly. There was no clear-cut explanation for the nerve injuries, but it must not be forgotten that the pressure in the cuff can easily be raised by an assistant casually resting an elbow on it, or from the pressure effect of a small, firm sandbag when the thigh is positioned on it. In Guanche's case, there was a large bruise on the posterior surface of the thigh where the tourniquet had been applied.

The pathology of tourniquet paralysis was described in Chapter 2. It is a neurapraxia, a localised block with demyelination. Larger fibres are most susceptible to pressure. There is relative sparing of sensation compared with motor function. Small-diameter fibres are spared, which explains the preservation of pain and temperature sensation and autonomic function. Because of the localised nature of the pathology, most lesions heal spontaneously in less than six months and permanent deficits are rare.[7] The chance of complete recovery is excellent.[1] Sensory defects are usually minor and tend to recover more rapidly than motor deficits.

The main cause of tourniquet paralysis is excessive pressure. This is avoided easily if the apparatus has an accurate gauge. Faulty anaeroid gauges have been reported frequently.[8] Nevertheless, it must not be forgotten that neural tissue may sometimes be unusually susceptible to pressure.[9] There may be neuropathy due to rheumatoid arthritis, alcohol or diabetes. Wasting of muscles may reduce the protection provided by muscles. Most lesions occur in the upper limb, where muscle bulk is less. According to Saunders and colleagues, nerve injuries following the use of inflatable cuffs on the lower limb are more common than is generally thought.[10] Postoperative weakness of the quadriceps may be due to pressure on the femoral nerve and not simply disuse atrophy. Saunders and colleagues followed 48 consecutive patients after arthrotomy with postoperative electromyography (EMG) of the quadriceps muscles. In cases where the duration of surgery exceeded one hour, EMG changes were as high as 85%. Abnormal EMGs have also been noted in 72% of patients following menisectomy 10–45 days after operation.[11] Perhaps the EMG changes and associated postoperative weakness have less significance in elderly or sedentary patients. The changes are much more important for active patients, especially athletes who need to become fully fit as rapidly as possible.

The effect on the strength of the leg was studied recently in a prospective, double-blind, randomised trial of 48 patients who had an anterior cruciate ligament reconstruction using an autologous graft from the patellar ligament.[12] The patients were randomised to having a tourniquet applied for the operation or to not having a tourniquet applied. The preliminary measurements were made one week before surgery. The average tourniquet time was 85±7 minutes (range 51–114) at 300 mm Hg. Anterior cruciate ligament reconstruction resulted in a significant decrease in thigh and calf girth and dorsiflexion and plantar flexion strength measured isometrically three weeks after operation in both groups. The patients who had tourniquets applied had a greater decrease in thigh girth than the control group. The use of a tourniquet had no effect on the strength of the quadriceps at six months, measured isokinetically at 60 degrees per second, with the patient seated. It was concluded that use of a tourniquet for less than 114 minutes had no effect on the strength of the lower limb after surgery.

The cases described so far have occurred after tourniquet times that vary from 28 minutes to two hours and 45 minutes.[13] The duration of ischaemia does not appear to be relevant to the occurrence of the nerve lesion, which is primarily the result of compression. Variations in time are related to differences in the magnitude of the deforming force and the internal structure of the nerve at the site of compression.[14] The radial nerve is the most vulnerable, followed by the median and ulnar nerves. The radial nerve is in the spiral groove adjacent to the humerus and therefore at risk of compression. Disturbances of sweating and causalgia have been described,[7] but this is rare.

A characteristic of the nerve lesion described in Chapter 2 is the relatively short duration of compression required to produce it. Experimentally, Rudge and colleagues produced a demyelinating block in the anterior tibial nerve of a baboon in one hour.[15] They stressed the value of electrophysiological studies for following progress in cases of tourniquet palsy.

There should be no difficulty in the diagnosis of tourniquet palsy. Confusion may occur rarely when the operative field is near a main nerve trunk or when the lesion has been undetected for a few days. As a rule, the sensory changes pass rapidly, whereas the motor symptoms last much longer. It is this dissociation between motor and sensory symptoms that helps to differentiate between a true division of one or more nerves.[3] In any event, the prognosis is good.

5.2 Damage to Muscle

5.2.1 Rhabdomyolysis

Sublethal damage to muscle is common and recovers rapidly (see Chapter 2). Rhabdomyolysis, the destruction of skeletal muscle, may occur occasionally. High levels of myoglobin result in acute renal failure. This situation is analogous to the crush syndrome first described by Bywaters and Beall in 1941, which resulted from falling masonry in the Battle of Britain.[16] It is rare following the use of a tourniquet, and only five cases have been recorded. The tourniquet time varies from 45 minutes in a case of burns[17] to 4.5 hours.[18]

Many of the clinical features are non-specific, but pyrexia, pain and tenderness at the site where the tourniquet cuff was applied, oedema, haemorrhagic discoloration, and oliguria are very suggestive of the diagnosis. It may follow severe compartment syndrome. Diagnosis is confirmed by a spot urine or serum myoglobin level.

Other features are cloudy urine, and significant elevation of serum creatinine phosphokinase and lactate dehydrogenase. The serum creatine, urea, urate and phosphate and potassium levels are raised, whereas sodium and calcium concentrates fall. Myoglobin is deposited in the distal convoluted tubule, ultimately causing occlusion. This may precipitate renal failure, but other factors such as anoxic renal tubules may be secondary. The treatment should be undertaken with a renal physician. In severe cases, haemodialysis or peritoneal dialysis may be necessary.

Myoglobin is released after the routine use of a tourniquet. The concentration in the plasma was assessed both before and up to 68 hours after release of the tourniquet in 27 patients who had elective operations with no incisions into skeletal muscle. A control group underwent the same type of surgery but without a tourniquet. There was minimal elevation of myoglobin values after 65 and 90 minutes of ischaemia and a marked elevation after 150 minutes. Maximum values were reached after eight to ten hours, falling to preoperative values after 50–60 hours. In this investigation, the disappearance of myoglobin took longer than after myocardial infarction.[19]

The reported clinical cases have included a 73-year-old man with severe osteo-arthritis of the hips and knees.[20] He developed symptoms after a total knee replacement with a well-padded pneumatic tourniquet on the mid-thigh. His past medical history included angina, hypertension and cardiac failure. His serum creatine kinase reached 16 000 IU (normal = 250 IU). After initial treatment with intravenous fluids and then high doses of diuretics and renal-dose dopamine, the patient's renal function returned to normal.

5.2.2 Compartment Syndrome

Use of a pneumatic tourniquet experimentally in dogs has been effective in producing a compartment syndrome in the fascial compartments distal to the site of the tourniquet application by creating post-ischaemic oedema of the muscles. Mubarak and Hargens found that tissue pressure rose above arterial diastolic pressure in 50% of hind limbs of dogs exposed to six hours of ischaemia after release of the tourniquet.[21] Swelling of the muscle increased the tissue pressure. Capillary blood flow was occluded by the high tissue pressure. These experimental conditions do not occur in clinical practice, but compartment syndromes have been reported rarely, usually with prolonged tourniquet times.

Using baboons, Mars and Brock-Utne showed that release of a tourniquet after it had been applied to the upper arm at a pressure of 100 mm Hg above systolic pressure for 90 minutes resulted in a transient increase in intracompartmental pressure of less than 30 minutes duration, in both bandaged and unbandaged limbs.[22] This was followed by a fall in intracompartmental pressure for up to three hours. The authors concluded that under normal circumstances, the release of a tourniquet and the ensuing hyperaemia do not appear to put the limb at risk of developing compartment syndrome.

A case of transient compartment syndrome resulting from venous congestion has been described.[23] During the procedure to internally fix a fractured proximal phalanx of the right index finger of an obese, hypertensive (blood pressure 160/90 mm Hg) patient, the procedure was complicated by venous bleeding. The pressure in the cuff fell to 80 mm Hg 30 minutes after the cuff was inflated. The cuff was reinflated to 280 mm Hg, but the venous ooze persisted. The tourniquet was deflated completely after 1.5 hours for 20 minutes. The air reservoir was changed and the cuff was reinflated to 300 mm Hg. The procedure was completed after a total tourniquet time of two hours and 35 minutes. When the hand was dressed at the end of the operation, the forearm flexor compartment was noted to be tense and rigid. The area of arm beneath the tourniquet was ecchymotic, and both the arm and forearm distal to the tourniquet were covered with petechiae. It was necessary to monitor the flexor compartment pressure using the technique of Whitesides and colleagues 8 and 10 cm distal to the antecubital fossa. Although these pressures were initially 50 and 55 mg Hg, respectively, they then decreased gradually over the next four hours to 15 mm Hg so that it was not necessary to decompress the forearm. The patient was discharged after 24 hours. After a week, the petechiae were still not resolved fully, but the muscular compartments of the forearm remained soft and there were no clinical signs of ischaemic contracture.

A venous tourniquet that does not allow blood out of the limb but does not limit arterial inflow is a potentially dangerous situation and may, as seen above, result in compartment syndrome The author has seen a single case in a young, fit man with muscular thighs who, while having a patellar fracture repaired, developed a gross compartment syndrome of the leg affecting all three compartments because of a venous tourniquet. After decompression, rhabdomyolysis followed; despite treatment in a renal unit, eventually the patient had to have an above-knee amputation.

A compartment syndrome of the arm where the tourniquet was applied has been reported.[24] The patient, a 29-year-old woman, had an interfascicular dissection of the right median nerve in the distal forearm and palm for fibrofatty infiltration of the nerve, with the use of a dissecting microscope. The tourniquet was applied and released on four occasions during the course of the operation, which took 12.5 hours. There were four breathing periods of 15 minutes, and the total tourniquet time was 655 minutes. The periods for which the tourniquet was inflated ranged in length from 95 to 140 minutes. Twelve hours after the operation, the patient had severe pain and swelling of the arm. There was a tense circumferential swelling of the right arm from the elbow to the shoulder, with a few small blisters at the site where the tourniquet had been applied. The forearm and hand were soft and not swollen. There was no pain on passive stretching of the digital flexors, but passive extension of the elbow caused severe pain in the arm. The intracompartmental pressure in the arm measured by the needle and manometer method of Whiteside was 70 mm Hg anteriorly and 50 mm Hg posteriorly. A fasciotomy was done through an incision over the medial intermuscular septum from the shoulder to the elbow. The compartment pressure dropped to 30 mm Hg in the anterior compartment of the forearm, and further fasciotomy was not considered necessary. There was an immediate and dramatic relief of the intense pain in the arm. One week later, delayed primary closure of the fasciotomy incision was carried out. There was no subsequent loss of neuromuscular function.

This case illustrates the relative ineffective outcome of breathing periods and considerably exceeded the safe period of an uninterrupted tourniquet time of three hours. Nowadays, if a prolonged operation is planned, one must consider supplementary techniques to protect the limb, such as preoperative cooling or pharmacological means. Three hours still remains a safe upper limit.

There is a report from Finland of two patients who developed severe compartment syndrome of the lower limb after surgery under a bloodless field for one hour and 25 minutes and 43 minutes, respectively, with reasonable tourniquet pressures.[25] Both patients required fasciotomies as an emergency procedure shortly after their initial operations. The first patient had a trimalleolar fracture of her ankle; the second had an elective exploration of his right Achilles tendon. Symptoms developed rapidly after the operations.

A report from Hong Kong describes a case in which compartment syndrome and tourniquet paralysis occurred simultaneously.[26] This provided a test of diagnostic acumen. The patient, a 26-year-old male, had a closed common trimalleolar fracture of the left ankle treated by open reduction and internal fixation. The tourniquet was applied to the thigh at a pressure of 450 mm Hg. The total tourniquet time was three hours and 15 minutes, but after the first two hours the tourniquet was deflated for 25 minutes and then reinflated. Postoperatively, the patient was found to have complete motor paralysis and almost complete sensory loss below the knee. Passive movement of the toes did not cause pain. A diagnosis of tourniquet paralysis was made. The pneumatic tourniquet and pressure gauge were checked and were in good order.

About 30 hours after the operation, the patient complained of severe pain in the front of the leg and a burning sensation in the sole of the foot. Active movements of the toes were detected for the first time. Passive movements produced severe pain in the anterior tibial compartment. Sensation to pinprick and light touch over the lower leg were still absent.

Emergency open fasciotomies of the anterior lateral and superficial posterior compartments were performed. The muscle in the anterior compartment was pale, with diminished contractibility; the other compartments were not under tension. Subsequently, debridement of the long toe extensors and tibialis anterior muscle was required because of necrosis. Three months after the fracture had healed, anterior transfer of the tibialis posterior tendon was used for correction of the drop foot.

The association of tourniquet paralysis and compartment syndrome is very rare and prompt diagnosis in this unusual situation is essentially based on clinical evidence.

In conclusion, the most likely cause of a postoperative compartment syndrome is the application of a tight, unyielding bandage or plaster after the release of the tourniquet.

5.3 Vascular Complications

A tourniquet should only be applied to a limb with a normal blood supply. Careful preoperative assessment of the circulation should be made of all patients having operations under tourniquet, especially on the lower limb. It is important to palpate the pedal pulses, assess the capillary filling time, and note the state of the skin and nails. Brittle, dry nails, shining, scaly skin, and loss of hairs indicate poor circulatory nutrition. The presence of varicose veins is of importance in relation to postoperative deep vein thrombosis and swelling. If pedal pulses are absent, then measurement of the ankle/brachial index (ABI) is essential. Using a Doppler probe, the blood pressure at the ankle is compared with the reading at the elbow; in normal circumstances, the ratio should be 1. If there is any doubt about the circulation, the opinion of a vascular surgeon is required. The application of a tourniquet to a limb with atheromatous vessels, commonly the superficial femoral artery, may result in poor wound healing and sepsis, ultimately requiring amputation (Figures 5.1 and 5.2).

A tourniquet should never be applied to a limb that has had an arterial prosthesis inserted .The implant is insufficiently elastic to dilate after release of the tourniquet and collateral circulation is likely to be defective.[9]

Fortunately, the incidence of arterial complications following total knee arthroplasty is lower than might be expected, particularly considering the proximity of the vessels to the knee joint in both flexion and extension.[27] Insall and Windsor state that the preoperative absence of peripheral pulses has not been regarded as a contraindication to surgery, provided that the capillary circulation is adequate.[28] In their experience, seven cases of arterial compromise occurred in more than 5000 arthroplasties, three resulting in amputation. Avoidance of a tourniquet may have prevented most, if not all, complications (see below). If a tourniquet is not used, bleeding can be profuse and troublesome and may compromise fixation when cement is used. Insall and Windsor recommend preoperative assessment by a vascular surgeon for those cases where there is doubt about the circulation. Acute vascular insufficiency following a total knee replacement may be caused either by direct injury to a major vessel or by thrombosis in an intact but diseased vascular system.

Rand, working at the Mayo Clinic, reported three cases of arterial injury associated with total knee arthroplasty in a series of 9022 patients during the period 1971–86.[29] He suggested that pre-existing arterial disease and correction of extensive flexion contractures appeared to be predisposing factors.

In a survey of the members of the British Association for Surgery of the Knee, there were three cases due to direct injury. One resulted in a false aneurysm.[30] There are several reports of similar occurrences. These three patients made a good recovery after corrective surgery. The outcome following thrombosis of an artery is different. Of the 11 patients in this survey, two died soon after surgery. Six required amputation, one had persistent symptoms and died two years later, and only two were reported to have recovered after vascular surgery. McAuley and colleagues suggested that the problem could be a disruptive external force applied to chronically diseased vessels.[31] Tethering of the proximal superficial femoral artery with stretching of the distal vessel may be responsible. Similarly, Rush and colleagues suggested that the pressure of the tourniquet may damage atheromatous vessels, causing fractures of plaques.[32] Lack of blood flow because of the tourniquet could then lead to thrombosis. Correction of a flexion deformity can result in a traction injury to the vessels. Stretching of atheromatous vessels may cause initial disruption and subsequent thrombosis. Due to calcification, the vessels may be incompressible, even when the cuff is inflated to the maximum. This situation is only likely to occur in elderly patients, and the presence of calcified vessels on plain radiographs should be a warning.[33, 34] In patients who require a total knee replacement and are

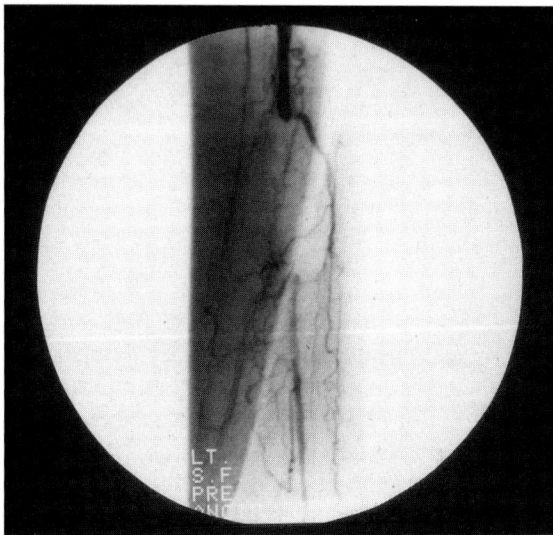

Figure 5.1 Arteriogram of a patient who had a dusky, cyanosed great toe after a Kellers' operation. Note the narrowed femoral artery.

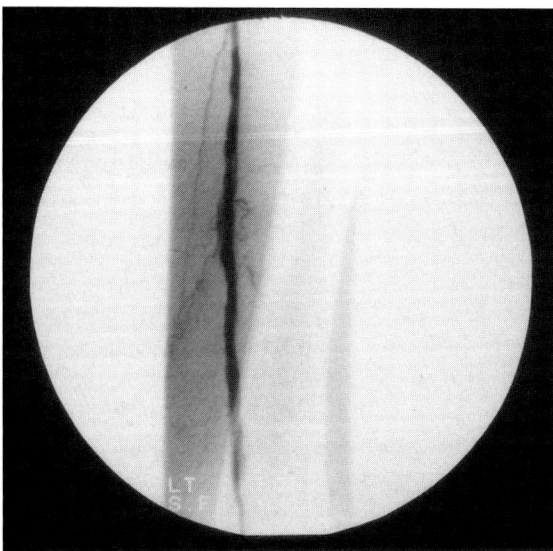

Figure 5.2 Arteriogram in the same patient as in Figure 5.1 after angioplasty had produced a pink toe. The use of a tourniquet on this patient was contraindicated. Always check the pulses.

not suitable for the use of a tourniquet, the operation can be done without a tourniquet.

Abdel-Salem and Eyres reported a controlled trial in a series of patients undergoing knee-replacement surgery.[35] Eighty patients were allocated randomly to two groups: operation with or without a tourniquet. The patients were all operated on by the same surgeon using the same prosthesis. There was no significant difference between the two groups in operating time or total blood loss. Postoperative pain was less in the patients in whom a tourniquet had not been used. They achieved straight leg raising and knee flexion earlier and had fewer superficial wound infections and deep vein thrombosis than the controls. Another prospective trial in 77 patients found similar results, but there was no difference in the incidence of wound complications or deep vein thrombosis between the two groups of patients.[36]

A prospective study was undertaken on the blood flow of 44 patients who were having total knee replacements under tourniquet control and who had no evidence of peripheral vascular disease.[37] The ABI did not alter after operation, and there were no changes in arterial waveforms. None of the limbs studied had an ABI below 0.87. Furthermore, none of the three limbs with ABI below 1 preoperatively showed any deterioration after operation. Doppler velocity waveforms, which are considered a more sensitive index of stenosis, were unchanged .The authors considered that the preoperative assessment should include duplex scanning as well as ABI measurements. Their final conclusion was that unless there is clinical evidence of peripheral vascular disease, then total knee replacement under a tourniquet is unlikely to cause ischaemic complications.

Traumatic arteriovenous fistulae with a false aneurysm of the inferior medial genicular artery have been reported following arthroplasty of the knee. Both cases were diagnosed within the first two months following surgery.[38] Both patients developed swellings in the regions of the incisions associated with a pulsatile swelling and audible bruit. The diagnosis was confirmed by arteriography. Surgical excision with ligation of the inferior medial genicular artery was effective in the relief of symptoms. Strict haemostasis after release of the tourniquet at the end of the operation should prevent this.

Giannestras and colleagues describe how an atheromatous plaque was displaced in the left superficial femoral artery following use of a tourniquet on the thigh for a bunion operation.[39] The foot remained pale when the tourniquet was deflated. The plaque was removed through an arteriotomy after an arteriogram had been performed. The tourniquet pressure used was 500 mg Hg – rather high and a possible factor – but there was no mention of the patient's blood pressure. The patient's subsequent course was uncomplicated.

Vessels in the foot may also be damaged at operation but pass unnoticed at the time. Webb Jones described three cases where aneurysms had developed after triple arthrodesis.[40] Scott recorded the formation of an aneurysm of the peroneal artery after an operation on the ankle through a posterolateral approach.[41]

It is the surgeon's duty to routinely inspect carefully the exposed digits after the tourniquet has been released in the operation theatre to ensure that there has been return of normal circulation. If there is any doubt about a digit, the bandages may need to be removed and reapplied. It is also important to continue to observe the circulation for the first 12–24 hours.

5.4 Damage to Skin

Damage to the skin was mentioned in Chapter 2. The most common problem is burns of the skin. Children appear to be particularly susceptible. Such burns have been appreciated for many years: McElvenny drew attention to them in 1945.[42] There are at least six references to chemical burns under a tourniquet, and the complication cannot be regarded as inconsequentially rare. It is discussed specifically in *Campbell's Operative Orthopaedics*.[43] Burns occur when the padding under the tourniquet becomes soaked by the antiseptic solution used to paint the skin. Aqueous solutions are not recorded as causing burns, and proprietary antibacterial agents are not responsible, except in specific allergic reactions, which are rare and result in skin irritation wherever applied. Alcohol-based solutions appear to be the most likely cause. The burns are due to prolonged contact of alcohol-based solutions since evaporation is prevented under the tourniquet (Figure 5.3).

These burns are easy to prevent using one of three methods. First, the skin preparation can be applied well distally to the tourniquet in operations below the knee or elbow. Second, the solutions should not be applied too liberally, as this promotes spillage and trickling towards the tourniquet. Finally, if the skin has to be prepared right up to the tourniquet, then it must be positively occluded from the prepared area for operation by using a drape with a rubber membrane, as is used frequently in knee surgery, or a drape with an adhesive edge stuck to the skin; the latter is the safest method.

A friction burn to the thigh has been described in a 48-year-old Caucasian man who underwent a second-stage knee replacement following revision for an infected prosthesis.[44] After skin preparation with aqueous chlorhexidine, the tourniquet was sealed off from the operation site by an adhesive drape. At the end of the operation, the tourniquet was found to have overrun the wool padding with almost half of its width and was lying in direct skin contact. The whole complex had slipped down the thigh by about 10 cm. The wool padding was not found to be soiled with blood or fluid. On the first postoperative day, the patient developed almost circumferential blisters on the thigh. It was presumed that the movement of fully inflated tourniquet over the base skin due to slippage led to friction burns. It was thought that the tourniquet had not been tied tightly enough before inflation.

5.5 Post-tourniquet Syndrome

This condition, according to Bruner, is the most common but least appreciated morbidity associated with the use of tourniquets.[45] In my experience, however, it is

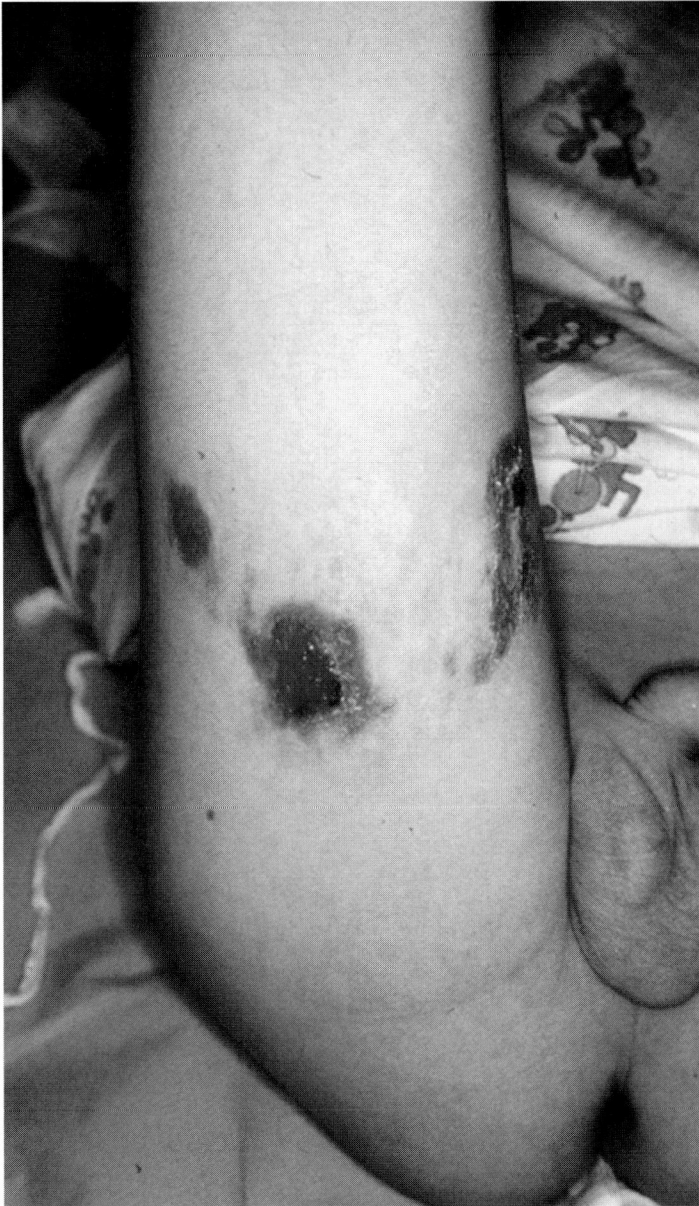

Figure 5.3 Typical circumferential burn occurring under a tourniquet. This painful lesion is easily prevented.

rare. The combined effect of muscle ischaemia, oedema, and microvascular congestion leads to a syndrome characterised by stiffness, pallor, weakness but not paralysis, and subjective numbness without anaesthesia. It probably represents the effects of a situation in which the upper limits of tissue tolerance have been reached, and it does not occur with relatively short periods of ischaemia of less than two hours.

5.6 Potential of Cross-infection During Peripheral Venous Access by Contamination of Tourniquets

Venepuncture for blood tests and intravenous cannulation are the most common invasive procedures carried out in hospitals. The usual method for providing venous stasis is the application of a reusable tourniquet. The use of such tourniquets in many patients and many wards contravenes the basic principles of infection control. One study has revealed a substantial reservoir of potentially pathogenic bacteria on these tourniquets, which can be transmitted from patient to patient on the hands of staff.[46] Reusable tourniquets have been shown to be potential fomites. Since it is impossible to disinfect reusable tourniquets (they are not made of durable material), the use of disposable tourniquets is recommended.

References

1 Speigel, IJ, Lewin, P (1943). Tourniquet paralysis. Analysis of three cases of surgically proved peripheral nerve damage following use of a rubber tourniquet. *Journal of the American Medical Association* **129**: 432–435.

2 Putnam, JJ (1888). Peripheral paralysis following use of a rubber tourniquet. *Boston Medical and Surgical Journal* **199**: 1888.

3 Eckhoff, NI (1931). Tourniquet paralysis. *Lancet* **2**: 343–345.

4 Middleton, RWD, Varian, JP. Tourniquet paralysis (1974). *Australia and New Zealand Journal of Surgery* **44**: 124–128.

5 Rorabeck, CH, Kennedy, JC (1980). Tourniquet induced nerve ischaemia complicating knee ligament surgery. *American Journal of Sports Medicine* **8**: 98–102.

6 Guanche, CJ (1995). Tourniquet-induced tibial nerve palsy complicating anterior cruciate reconstruction. *Journal of Arthroscopic and Related Surgery* **11**: 620–622.

7 Bolton, CF, McFarlane, RM (1978). Human pneumatic tourniquet paralysis. *Neurology* **28**: 787–793.

8 Klenerman, L (1983). Tourniquet paralysis. *Journal of Bone and Joint Surgery* **65B**: 374–375.

9 Birch, R, Bonney, G, Wyn Parry, CB, eds (1998). *Surgical Disorders of the Peripheral Nerves*. London: Churchill Livingston, pp. 301–302.

10 Saunders, K, Louis, D, Weingarden, SI, Waylonis, GW (1979). Effect of tourniquet time on postoperative quadriceps function. *Clinical Orthopaedics and Related Research* **143**: 194–199.

11 Weingarden, SI, Louise, DL, Waylonis, GW (1979). Electromyographic changes in postmeniscectomy patients. *Journal of the American Medical Association* **241**: 1248–1250.

12 Nicholas, TJ, Tyler, TF, McHugh, MP, Gleim, GW (2001). Effect on leg strength of tourniquet use during anterior cruciate reconstruction: a prospective randomised study. *Journal of Arthroscopic and Related Surgery* **17**: 603–607.

13 Aho, K, Saino, K, Kienta, M, Varpanen, E (1983). Pneumatic tourniquet paralysis. *Journal of Bone and Joint Surgery* **65B**: 441–443.

14 Sunderland, S (1968). *Nerves and Nerve Injuries*. Edinburgh: E & S Livingstone, p. 141.

15 Rudge, P, Ochoa, J, Gilliatt, RW (1974). Acute peripheral nerve compression in the baboon. *Journal of Neurological Sciences* **23**: 403–420.

16 Bywaters, EGL, Beall, D (1941). Crush injuries with impairment of renal function. *British Medical Journal* **1**: 427–432.

17 Pfeiffer, PM (1986). Acute rhabdomyolysis. Possible role of tourniquet ischaemia. *Anaesthesia* **41**: 614–619.

18 Williams, JE, Tucker, DB, Read, JM (1983). Rhabdomyolysis – myoglobin. Consequences of prolonged tourniquet. *Journal of Foot Surgery* **22**: 52–56.

19 Jorgensen, HRI (1987). Myoglobin release after tourniquet ischaemia. *Acta Orthopaedica Scandinavica* **58**: 554–556.

20 Palmer, SH, Graham, G (1994). Tourniquet induced rhabdomyolysis after total knee replacement. *Annals of the Royal College of Surgeons of England* **76**: 416–417.

21 Mubarak, S, Hargens, A (1981). *Compartment Syndrome and Volkmann's Contracture.* Philadelphia: W.B. Saunders, p. 50.

22 Mars, M, Brock-Utne, JG (1991). The effect of tourniquet release on intra-compartmental pressure in the bandaged and unbandaged limb. *Journal of Hand Surgery* **16B**: 318–322.

23 O'Neil, D, Sheppard, JE (1989). Transient compartment syndrome of the forearm resulting from venous congestion from a tourniquet. *Journal of Hand Surgery* **14A**: 894–896.

24 Greene, TL, Dean, S (1983). Compartment syndrome of the arm – a complication of the pneumatic tourniquet. *Journal of Bone and Joint Surgery* **65A**: 270–273.

25 Hirvensalo, E, Tuomen, H, Lapensuo, M, Helio H (1992). Compartment syndrome of the lower limb caused by a tourniquet: a report of two cases. *Journal of Orthopaedic Trauma* **6**: 469–472.

26 Luk, KD, Pun, WK (1987). Unrecognised compartment syndrome with tourniquet palsy. *Journal of Bone and Limb Surgery* **69B**: 97–99.

27 Zaidi, SHA, Cobb, AG, Bentley, G (1995). Danger to popliteal artery in high tibial osteotomy. *Journal of Bone and Joint Surgery* **77B**: 384–386.

28 Insall, JN, Windsor, RE, eds (1993). *Surgery of the Knee*, 2nd edn. New York: Churchill Livingstone, p. 896.

29 Rand, JA (1987). Vascular complications of total knee arthroplasty. *Journal of Arthroplasty* **2**: 89–93.

30 Kumar, NS, Chapman, JA, Rawlins, I (1998). Vascular injuries in total knee arthroplasty. *Journal of Arthroplasty* **13**: 211–216.

31 McAuley, CE, Steed, DL, Webster, MW (1984). Arterial complications of knee replacement. *Archives of Surgery* **119**: 960–962.

32 Rush, J, Vidovich, H, Johnson, MA (1987). Arterial complications of knee replacement. *Journal of Bone and Joint Surgery* **69B**: 400–406.

33 Klenerman, L, Lewis, JD (1976). Incompressible vessels. *Lancet* **1**: 811–812.

34 Jeyaseelan, S, Stevenson, TM, Pfitzner, J (1981). Tourniquet failure and arterial calcification. *Anaesthesia* **36**: 48–50.

35 Abdel-Salaam, A, Eyres, KA (1995). Effects of tourniquet during total knee arthroplasty. *Journal of Bone and Joint Surgery* **77B**: 250–253.

36 Wakenkar, HM, Nicholl, JE, Koka, R, D'Arcy, J (1999). The tourniquet in knee arthroplasty. *Journal of Bone and Joint Surgery* **81B**: 30–33.

37 Scriven, MW, Fligelstone, LJ, Oshodi, TO, et al. (1996). The influence of total knee arthroplasty on lower limb blood flow. *Journal of the Royal College of Surgeons of Edinburgh* **41**: 323–324.

38 Dennis, DA, Newmann, RD, Toma, P, et al. (1987). Arteriovenous fistula with false aneurysm of the inferior geniculate artery. *Clinical Orthopaedics and Related Research* **222**: 255–259.

39 Giannestras, NJ, Cranley, JJ, Lentz, M (1977). Occlusion of tibial artery after a foot operation under tourniquet. *Journal of Bone and Joint Surgery* **59A**: 682–683.

40 Webb Jones, A (1955). Aneurysm after foot stabilisation. *Journal of Bone and Joint Surgery* **37B**: 440–442.

41 Scott, JH (1955). Traumatic aneurysm of the peroneal artery. *Journal of Bone and Joint Surgery* **37B**: 438–439.

42 McElvenny, RT (1945). The tourniquet. Its clinical application. *American Journal of Surgery* **LXIX**: 94–106

43 Crenshaw, A, ed. (1987). *Cambell's Operative Orthopaedics*, Vol. 1, 7th edn. St Louis: CV Mosby, p. 111.

44 Choudhary, S, Koshy, C, Ahmed, J, Evans, J (1998). Friction burns to the thigh caused by tourniquet. *British Journal of Plastic Surgery* **51**: 142–143.

45 Bruner, JM (1951). Safety factors in the use of the pneumatic tourniquet in the hand. *Journal of Bone and Joint Surgery* **33A**: 221–224.

46 Golder, M, Chan, CLH, O'Shea, S, et al. (2000). Potential risk of cross-infection during peripheral venous access by contamination of tourniquets. *Lancet* **355**: 44.

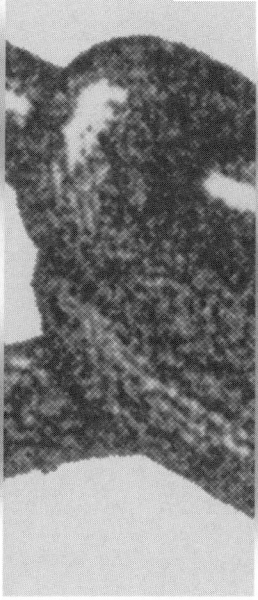

Chapter 6
The Tourniquet Used for Anaesthesia

THIS CHAPTER DISCUSSES intravenous regional anaesthesia and digital tourniquets.

6.1 Intravenous Regional Anaesthesia

In 1908, August Karl Gustav Bier (1851–1949; Figure 6.1), first assistant to Johann Frederick August von Esmarch at the time, devised an effective method of bringing about complete anaesthesia and motor paralysis of a limb. J. Leonard Corning had, in 1895, published the results of experiments of the effects of how the use of a tourniquet after subcutaneous injection of five minims of cocaine into the forearm prolonged and intensified the anaesthesia.[1] If the injection was carried out after exsanguination and compression, there was little diffusion of the anaesthetic and a reduction in the number of nerve filaments exposed to the influence of the solution. If the drug was injected a few moments before exsanguination and the

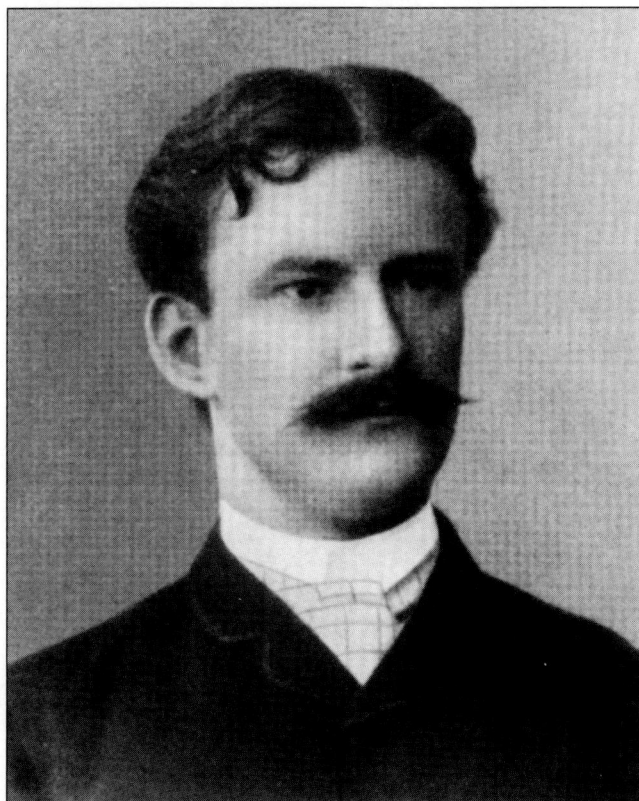

Figure 6.1 August Bier in his youth. Reprinted with permission from the Wellcome Library, London.

application of the tourniquet, a sufficient saturation of the tissue was achieved to expose a large number of the nerve filaments to the solution. Corning suggested that this technique was applicable to surgery of the extremities. Bier, a pioneer of spinal anaesthesia, established this technique. It was cumbersome by modern standards. He injected a solution of procaine into a subcutaneous vein on a section of the forearm that was visible between two constricting bands and that had been rendered bloodless by an Esmarch bandage. A surgical cut-down was required to locate the vein. The injected solution permeated through the exposed section of the limb very quickly and produced what Bier called "direct vein anaesthesia" in 5–15 minutes. The anaesthesia lasted for as long as the upper constricting band was left in place. After its removal, sensation returned in a few minutes.

The development of techniques of regional anaesthesia followed that of drugs that could produce local anaesthesia. Gaedicke isolated cocaine in 1855. It was purified and named by Nieman in 1860 and first used as a local anaesthetic by Koller in 1864. Cocaine was used for infiltration anaesthesia and major nerve blocks, which were popularised by both Halsted and Crile. The systemic toxicity of cocaine limited its use as a local anaesthetic. The practice of regional blocks was enhanced greatly when procaine was synthesised by Einhorn in 1904. Braun went on to establish the use of procaine for regional anaesthesia.[2]

The technique did not become used widely, despite Bier's reports of its use with Esmarch bandages in 134 patients, including ten amputations, 37 resections, 12 sutures of bones, ten tendon transfers, two Dupuytren's contractures, and seven cases of extirpation of varicose veins. Bier first conceived the possibility of the method when he injected a solution of indigo carmine into the veins of an amputated limb.[3] He found that there was widespread diffusion of the dye. He considered that the anaesthesia was of two types: direct and indirect. Direct anaesthesia was due to infiltration of the fluid into the tissues and around the nerve filaments and occurred rapidly. A little later, because of blocking of the larger nerve trunks passing through the exsanguinated region, further anaesthesia occurred distally (indirect anaesthesia) Today, the mechanism remains open to dispute and a combination of theories may best explain the effects.

Despite Bier's report of none of 134 patients showing any ill effects, his technique appears to have been forgotten until 1963, when it was reintroduced by Holmes.[4] The technique was used on a limited scale but did not gain widespread popularity. There are a number of reasons for this[5]: the technique was cumbersome, requiring wrapping and unwrapping of Esmarch bandages in a precise manner; special equipment was required; and an operative procedure (cut-down) was used. It was Morrison in 1931 who first suggested a venepuncture and made the method more practicable.[6] Although Holmes used lignocaine, 0.5% prilocaine is now regarded as the drug of choice.[7] Only the 0.5% solution should be used, and the recommended dose is 3–4 mg/kg.

The method has now been refined. An intravenous cannula should be inserted into each hand. The limb should be exsanguinated before the tourniquet is inflated. This can be done by elevation and careful application of an Esmarch bandage, taking care not to dislodge the intravenous needle; alternatively, a pneumatic splint can be used.[8] With the tourniquet inflated, the local anaesthetic agent is injected slowly. A double cuff can be used proximally; once anaesthesia has been achieved, the upper cuff can be released after the lower one has been inflated. It must be remembered that a significantly higher pressure is necessary (systolic plus 100 mm Hg) for the double cuff because of its narrow width, although in this way the pain from the tourniquet cuff can be reduced.

There is no doubt that a single cuff is easier, less complicated, and safer to use (Figure 6.2). The effect of exsanguination is not completely clear. The most important reason for exsanguination is to collapse the vascular compartment of the limb, i.e. to empty the blood from the limb and allow the space to be taken up by local anaesthetic. Injection of the anaesthetic solution into a full vascular compartment will impair complete distribution through the distal part of the limb. With the tourniquet inflated, the vascular compartment is a closed space, and relative collapse of the compartment is necessary to be able to accommodate the injection of the solution. The blotchy areas of erythema that appear as the anaesthetic is injected result from residual blood forced into the skin. The appearance of these areas indicates wide distribution of the anaesthetic. They appear regardless of the method used for exsanguination and do not signify that one is to expect poor analgesia.

Intravenous regional anaesthesia is a potentially dangerous technique because of the possibility of injection into the systemic circulation. Precautions are required in all cases. All the equipment used must be checked for leaks. The patient must be prepared and starved. Drugs for resuscitation are required. Full monitoring of the cardiovascular system must be available. Rapid injection of local anaesthetic should be avoided, since it may force fluid past the tourniquet. The needle should be as far distal as possible, and not in the antecubital fossa. Caution is needed for hypertensive and arteriosclerotic patients, as the tourniquet may not completely compress the main vessels in the arm.

This technique should not be performed by the surgeon alone. An anaesthetist is required to ensure adequate supervision of the patient. Analgesia is usually complete within four to six minutes, continuing for up to 90 minutes. However, procedures lasting for more than half an hour become uncomfortable because of pain from the tourniquet. Early loss of cutaneous sensation to pinprick is a good guide to the

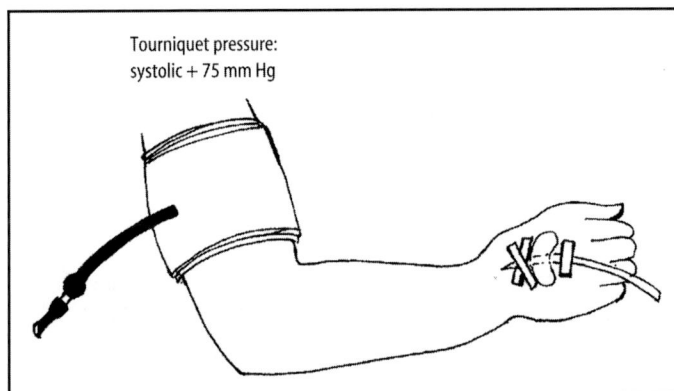

Tourniquet pressure:
systolic + 75 mm Hg

Figure 6.2 Diagram of a single cuff and intravenous needle after exsanguination. The intravenous needle is as far distal as possible. This is the simplest and safest technique.

effectiveness of the block. As muscle relaxation occurs, the limb should feel heavy to the patient.

This method is useful for distal fractures in the upper limb, ganglions and decompression of the median nerve. It is not used commonly for the lower limb, mainly because of the volume of local anaesthetic agent required.

After completion of the operation, the cuff should be deflated gradually in a step-wise manner to avoid a bolus injection of local anaesthetic. Sensation and motor power return after several minutes. The minimum tourniquet time suggested is 20 minutes to allow adequate diffusion into the ischaemic region.

The adverse effects of intravenous regional anaesthesia are due to accidental, sudden deflation of the cuff and deflation too soon after the injection of local anaesthetic. Sudden release results in a bolus of any unfixed local anaesthetic. Underinflation of the cuff will allow leakage to occur into the systemic circulation.

In 1982, in an editorial in the *British Medical Journal*, Margaret Heath noted that since 1979 the Scientific and Technical Branch of the Department of Health and Social Security in London had been informed of five deaths resulting directly from the use of intravenous regional analgesia.[9] The drug used was bupivacaine. In three of the most recent cases, it was found that the equipment was in good order but the cuff had been deflated when it should not have been.

The likelihood of direct intravenous injection during routine procedures has been underestimated. The effects of such a bolus are likely to be worse in frightened patients, as circulatory catecholamines will ensure that the maximum amount of the cardiac output reaches the brain and heart, which are the main target organs for toxicity. The recognition and treatment of toxic reactions are crucial. There is also the problem of individual low thresholds. Major side effects of using prilocaine have not been recorded in Britain. Prilocaine is the safest local anaesthetic for intravenous local anaesthesia. It is no longer available in North America in a form suitable for intravenous injection because of concern about methaemoglobinaemia, although this does not occur in the dosages used; lidocaine is commonly used in North America instead.[10]

6.2 Digital Tourniquets

When performing a minor procedure on a single digit, finger or toe, it is convenient to apply a tourniquet at the base of the digit rather than use a proximal tourniquet for the whole limb. A variety of techniques have been described. A common method is to wrap a soft rubber catheter or Penrose drain around the base of the finger or toe under tension and keep it in place with an artery forceps. Salem suggested a method that is now used commonly[11]: he cut off the finger of a disposable glove, removed the tip, stretched and applied it to the digit for operation, and rolled it proximally to form a ring at the base of the digit. This provides a satisfactory blood-less field. The ring can readily be cut and removed when the operation has been

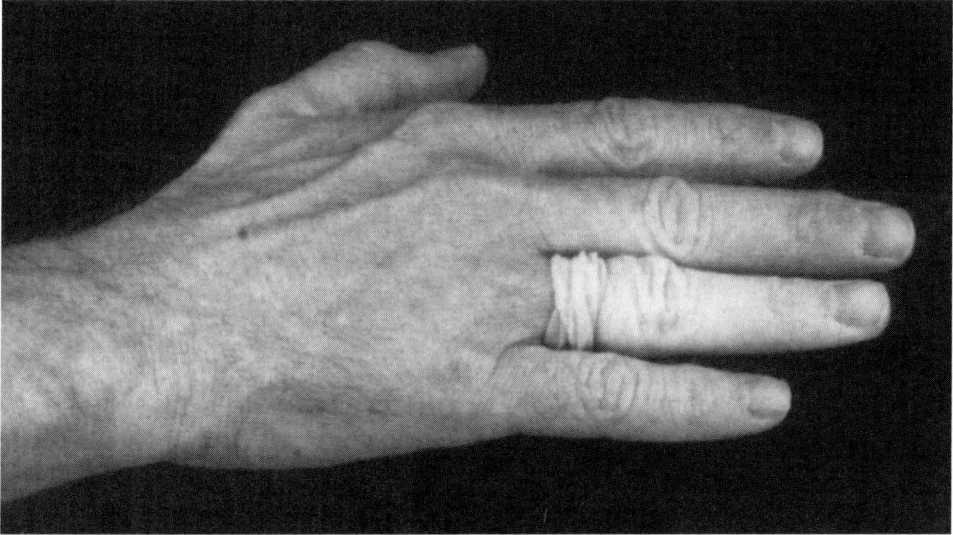

Figure 6.3 Salem's method of applying a digital tourniquet: (a) A finger from a rubber glove is rolled proximally.

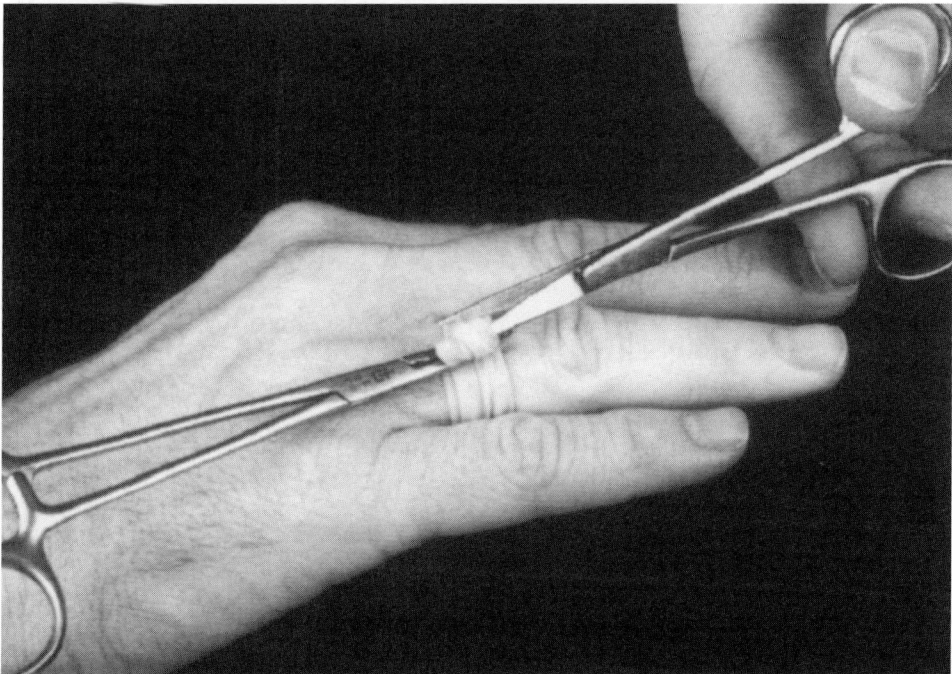

Figure 6.3 (b) The tourniquet is grasped in an artery clip.

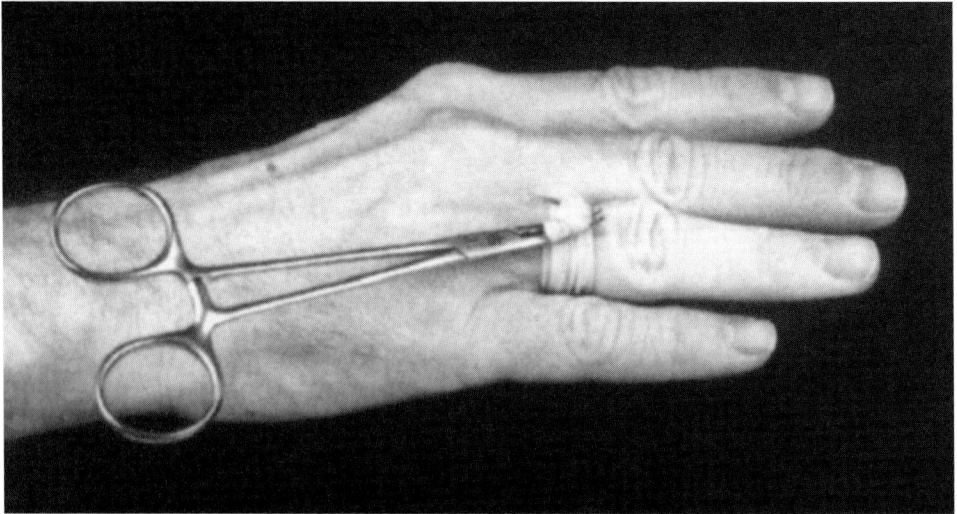

Figure 6.3 (c) The rubber ring is cut above the clip. Reproduced with permission from Elsevier Science from Smith, IM, Austin, OB, Knight, SL (2002). A simple and failsafe method for digital tourniquet. *Journal of Hand Surgery* 27B; 363–364.

completed. A recent modification suggests that the tourniquet should be gripped by an artery clip, with the handle pointing proximally.[12] The rubber ring is cut above the clip with scissors. This ensures that when the tourniquet is released, the danger of the tourniquet remaining in place is avoided (Figure 6.3). A study of the pressures involved using a miniature pressure transducer and digital strain indicator has shown that the Penrose drain generated highly variable pressure, often greater than 500 mg Hg.[13] In contrast, the rolled finger from a glove, in addition to producing exsanguination, uniformly generated pressures of less than 500 mg Hg, which is below the threshold required to produce nerve damage.

The main danger is that a digital tourniquet may be forgotten, covered with a dressing, and left to cause gangrene in the anaesthetised finger or toe (Figure 6.4). A rare case of ischaemia of the distal half of a finger has been reported, which recovered with treatment by intravenous infusion of low-molecular-weight dextrose, intravenous dipyridamole, and alcohol. The finger was packed in ice and the arm was warmed. The report was from a unit using a tourniquet for at least 1000 operations a year, and this was the first complication observed.[14]

6.3 Regional Sympathetic Blockade

For patients suffering complex regional pain syndrome (CRPS) type I (also known as reflex sympathetic dystrophy), a technique similar to intravenous regional anaesthesia has been used with a tourniquet in place.[15] A solution of 20 mg (for the upper limb) or 30 mg (for the leg) of guanethidine in normal saline is injected. The cuff is kept inflated for 15 minutes. This produces complete sympathetic blockade

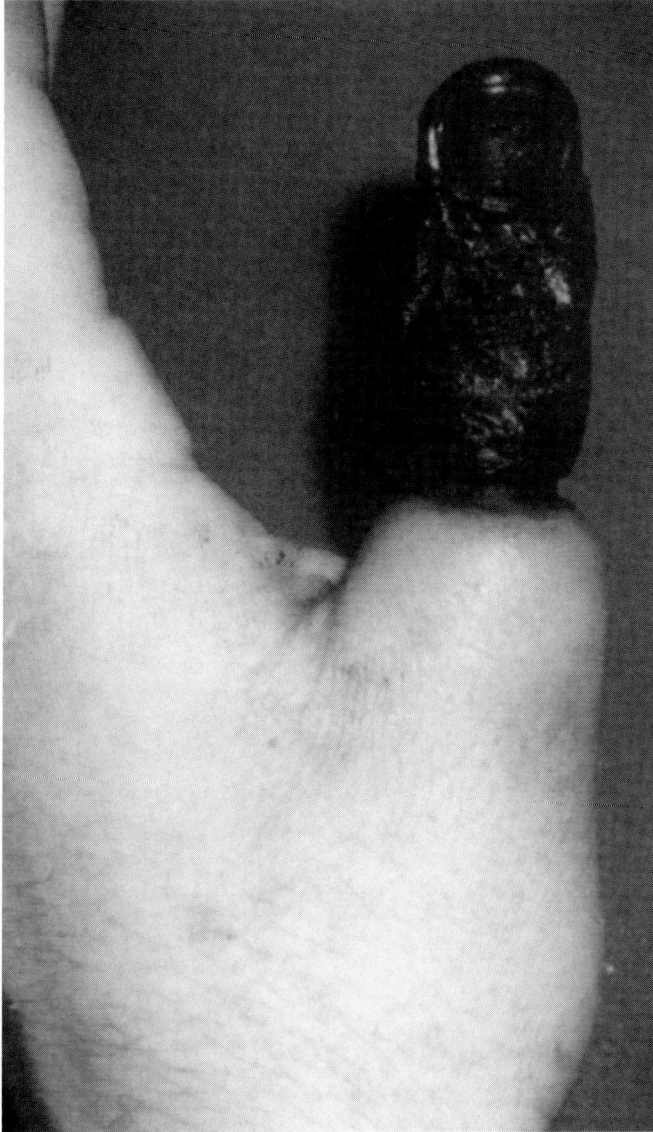

Figure 6.4 Gangrenous thumb after a digital tourniquet had been left in place for too long. Reproduced with permission from Elsevier Science from Smith, IM, Austin, OB, Knight, SL (2002). A simple and failsafe method for digital tourniquet. *Journal of Hand Surgery* 27B; 363–364.

for up to four days, reducing the pain in the affected limb and allowing active physiotherapy. Although this technique has been considered accepted practice for many years, recent work has shown that guanethidine offers no significant advantage in analgesia over a normal saline placebo block in the treatment of early CRPS type 1 of the hand after a fracture of the distal radius.[16] Guanethidine does not improve the outcome of this condition, and it may delay the resolution of vasomotor instability when compared with placebo.

References

1 Corning, JL (1895). Anaesthetic effects of the hydrochlorate of cocaine when subcutaneously injected. *New York Medical Journal* **42**; 317–319.
2 Hilgenhurst, G (1990). The Bier block after eighty years. *Regional Anaesthesia* **15**: 2–5.
3 Adams, RC (1944). *Intravenous Anaesthesia*. New York: Paul B. Hoeber, p. 111.
4 Holmes, CM (1963). Intravenous regional anaesthesia. *Lancet* **1**: 245–247.
5 Colbern, EC (1970). The Bier block for intravenous regional anaesthesia. Technique and literature review. *Anaesthesia and Analgesia* **49**: 935–940.
6 Morrison, JL (1931). Intravenous local anaesthesia. *British Journal of Surgery* **18**: 641–647.
7 Bader, AM, Concepion, M, Hurley, RJ, Arthur, GR (1998). Comparison of lidocaine and prilocaine for intravenous regional anaesthesia. *Anesthesiology* **69**: 409–412.
8 Winnie, AP, Ramamurthy, S ((1970.). Pneumatic exsanguination for intravenous regional anaesthesia. *Anesthesiology* **33**: 664–5.
9 Heath, M (1982). Deaths after intravenous regional anaesthesia. *British Medical Journal* **285**: 913–914.
10 Henderson, CL,Warriner, CB, McEwen, JA, Merrick, PM (1997). A North American survey of intravenous regional anaesthesia. *Anaesthesia and Analgesia* **85**: 853–863.
11 Salem, MZA (1973). Simple finger tourniquet. *British Medical Journal* **2**: 779.
12 Smith, IM, Austin, OB, Knight, SL (2002). A simple and fail safe method for digital tourniquet. *Journal of Hand Surgery* **27B**: 363–364.
13 Hixson, FP, Shafiroff, BB, Werner, FW, Palmer, AK (1986). Digital tourniquet a pressure study with relevance. *Journal of Hand Surgery* **11A**: 865–867.
14 Dove, AF, Clifford, RP (1982). Ischaemia after use of a finger tourniquet. *British Medical Journal* **284**: 1162–1163.
15 Hannington-Kiff, JG (1974). Intravenous regional sympathetic block with guanethidine. *Lancet* **i**: 1019–1020.
16 Livingstone, JA, Atkins, RM (2002). Intravenous regional blockade in the treatment of post-traumatic complex regional pain syndrome type 1 (algodystrophy) of the hand. *Journal of Bone and Joint Surgery* **84B**: 380–386.

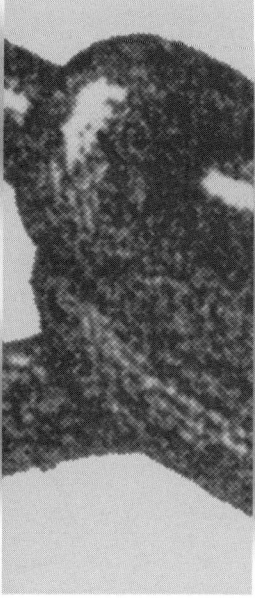

Chapter 7
Technology and Practice

THE PNEUMATIC TOURNIQUET includes a pressure source, pressure gauge, regulator and inflatable cuff (Figure 7.1). There are two types of tourniquet: those inflated by direct hand-pumping and those that are inflated "automatically" by the movement of a switch that controls an air or gas supply.[1] It is essential to ensure that the cuff is inflated rapidly to prevent venous congestion.

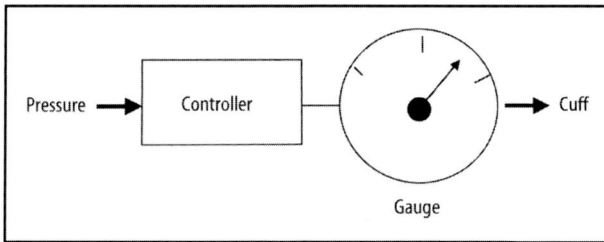

Figure 7.1 **Components of an automatic tourniquet control unit.** Reproduced with permission from Lippincott, Williams & Wilkins from Hurst, LN, Weiglein, O, Brown, WE, Campbell, GJ (1981). The pneumatic tourniquet: a biomechanical and electrophysiological study. *Plastic and Reconstructive Surgery* 648–652.

7.1 Design of the Tourniquet Cuff

Generally, the cuff is composed of one or two rectangular inflatable pneumatic bags made of rubber on plastic. These are enclosed in a cover of cloth or plastic, together with a firm backing sheet known as a spine (Figure 7.2). The pneumatic bags are inflated from a hand pump or a regulated source of compressed air via connecting tubes and links. A strapping mechanism is provided to retain the tourniquet in place on the arm or leg.

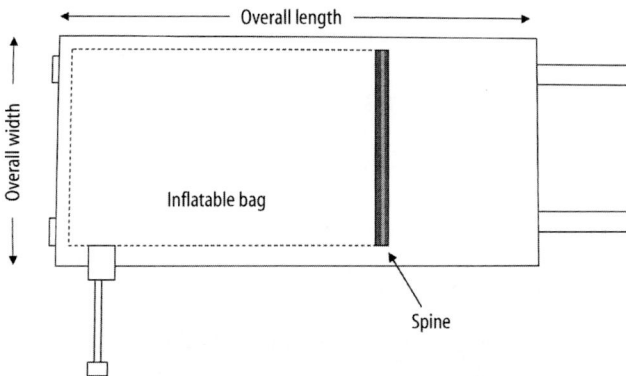

Figure 7.2 Diagram of a tourniquet cuff.

7.2 Hand-powered Tourniquets

A sphygmomanometer bulb or bicycle pump can be used for inflation. This type of tourniquet has the virtue of simplicity. It is not possible to preset a pressure. It is unlikely that accidental overinflation will occur since the tourniquet is inflated with a deliberate pumping action.

The pressure gauge is of an aneroid type (Figure 7.3). The gauge must be maintained carefully since it is vulnerable to knocks and is damaged readily. Displacement of the pin at the end of the range of pressure measurements has resulted in gross overinflation of the cuff.[2]

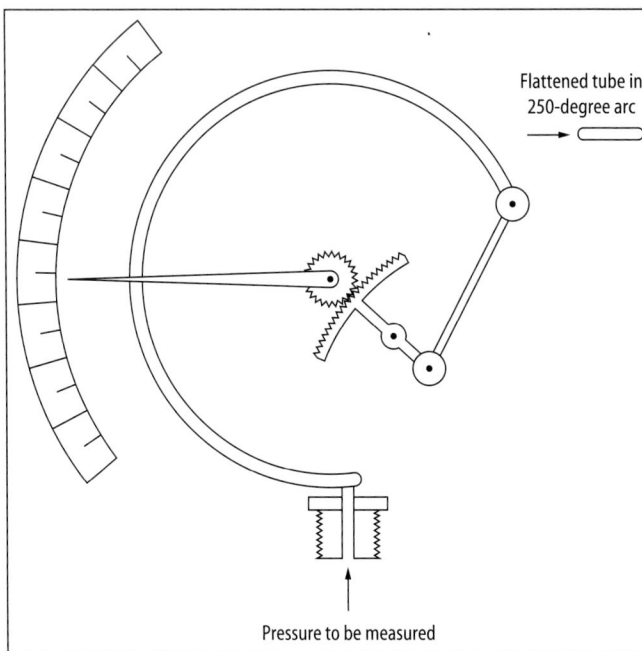

Flattened tube in 250-degree arc

Pressure to be measured

Figure 7.3 Diagram of a Bourdon gauge commonly used with tourniquet equipment. Reprinted with permission from the BMJ Publishing Group from Hallett, J (1983). Inaccurate tourniquet gauges. *British Medical Journal* 286: 1267.

7.3 Automatic Tourniquets

Development over the last 25 years has resulted in a variety of automatic systems now being available. Some use a self-contained gas source, such as a small cylinder of dichlorodifluoromethane or freon gas, to inflate the cuff. Others have an air reservoir that may be charged from a compressed air line. The machines can sometimes compensate for small leakages of pressure.

The most common tourniquet systems now available include automatic safety devices that operate from the main air supply or cylinders at a maximum pressure of 100 psi. A typical example is the Anetic Aid (Guiseley, Leeds, UK) APT Tourniquet.

This can be used from a piped service or from air cylinders. It has a dual-channel, self-compensating inflation capacity. The separate channels are indicated as A and B and are colour-coded. The hosing that supplies the cuff is also colour-coded to avoid confusion. Both channels can be used simultaneously, whilst remaining operated independently. Each channel has two secondary pressure gauges (Figure 7.4), one for preselection of the cuff pressure and the other showing actual cuff pressure on inflation using an aneroid gauge. Times are included automatically for each channel and are activated from the moment of inflation. On deflation, timing ceases but the record of the duration remains on display until the inflation switch is used again.

Also available are more advanced tourniquets with their own power supply for inflation, such as the AET Electronic Tourniquet (Anetic Aid) (Figures 7.5 and 7.6). This includes a microprocessor that performs self-calibration, displays elapsed inflation

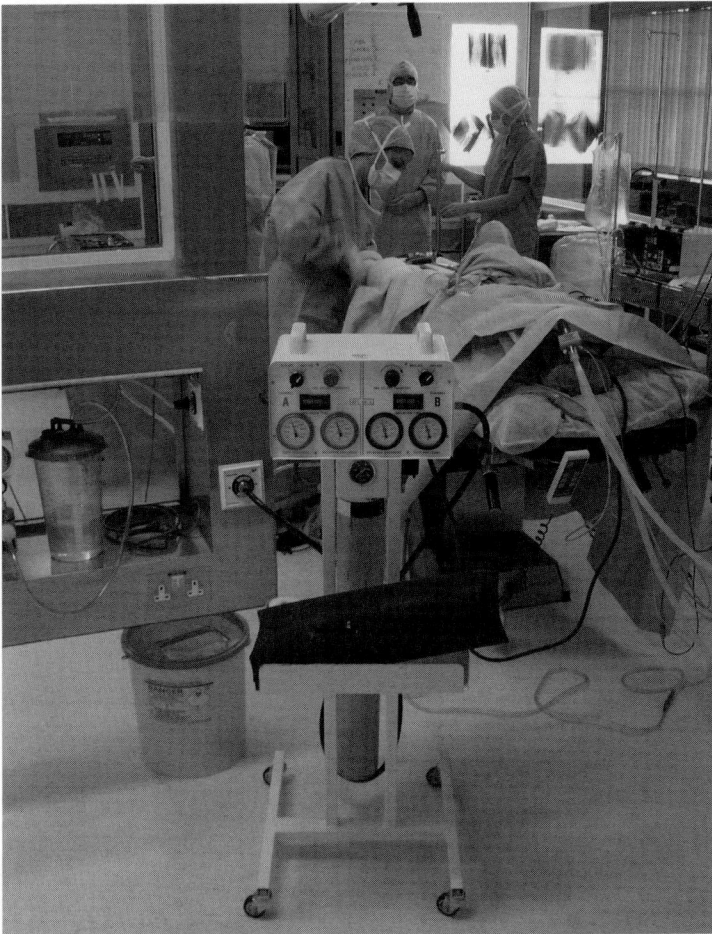

Figure 7.4 (a) Bilateral tourniquets in use in the theatre.

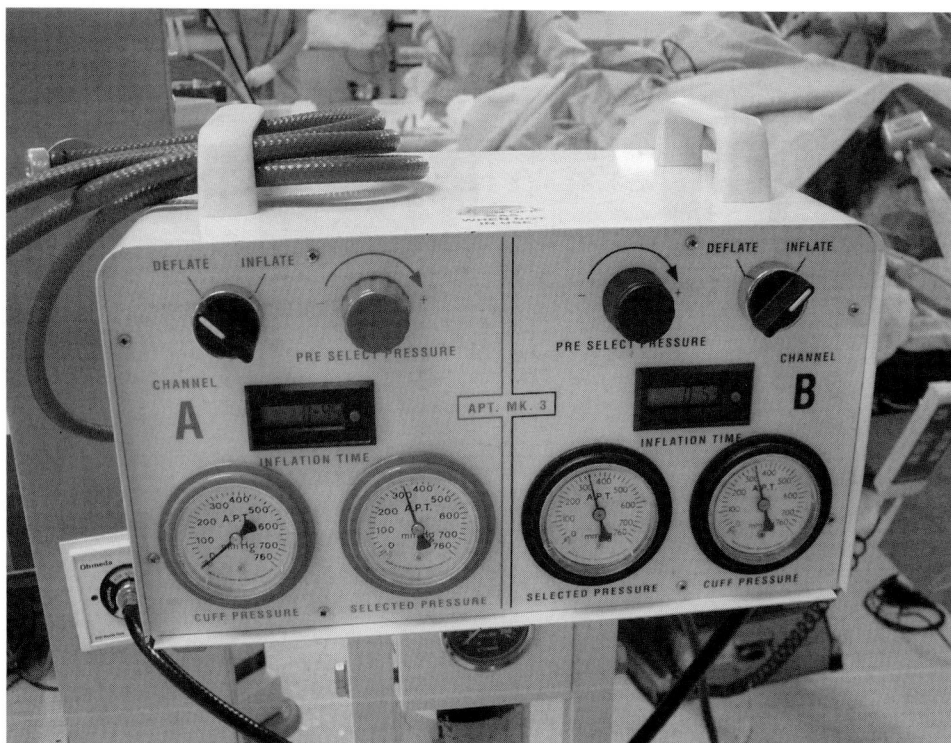

Figure 7.4 (b) Tourniquet linked to compressed air, showing close-up of dials: one tourniquet is inflated and the other has been deflated.

time, and sounds an alarm half-hourly. It uses an internal electrical pump to compress the ambient air, and pressure is shown on a microprocessor digital display. It can store the details of up to 20 applications, which can be recalled if necessary.

7.4 Safety Aspects

The safety aspects of tourniquets are summarised in a paper in the *American Operating Room Nurses Journal*.[3] All parts of the tourniquet should be checked before use to eliminate leaks from loose connectors, faulty tubing or the cuff bladder. A common source of leaks are worn O-rings, which help to seal the connection between the tourniquet and the tubes for inflation. The tourniquet apparatus must be treated with respect, as unnecessary jarring or bumping will damage the gauge and result in faulty readings. Routine and regular calibration of all tourniquets is mandatory. This can be done with a commercially available test gauge or a mercury column. A simple precaution is readily available at all times[4]: before the use of any tourniquet, the pressure gauge is set at 100 mm Hg and connected to the mercury manometer on the anaesthetic machine. The pressure in the tourniquet line is then released and the pressure on the mercury manometer is read. The procedure is then repeated

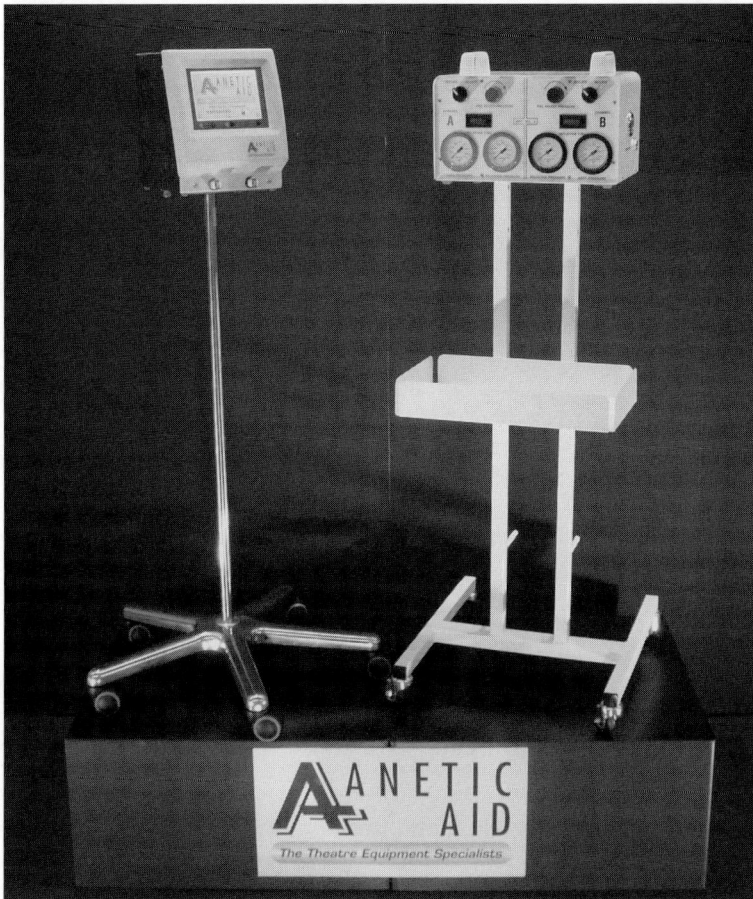

Figure 7.5 Two commonly used tourniquets: the left-hand tourniquet has a microprocessor, while the right-hand one needs to be connected to piped air or cylinders. Reprinted courtesy of Anetic Aid, Guiseley, Leeds, UK.

with the pressure gauge set at 200 mm Hg. Inaccurate gauges should be returned to the manufacturer. Inaccurate pressure gauges are one of the most common causes of pressure lesions in nerves (see Chapter 2).[5] Once a gauge becomes inaccurate, it cannot be readjusted and it must be replaced The Bourdon gauge will suffer from rough handling, and the flexibility of the metal coil will be altered with repeated use.[6]

The aneroid gauge may not always be at fault. Durkin and Crabtree reported a case in which the indicator needle on the pressure gauge could travel around the dial a second time, so that if the cuff was inflated quickly it might not be apparent that a reading of 250 mm Hg was actually representing a pressure of 1000 mg Hg.[2] This hazard could be avoided if all pressure gauges used for such purposes had a stop at the upper end of the scale. Cuff pressure within ±20 mm Hg of indicated dial pressure is acceptable.[6] The complete system should be leak-proof, with no change in pressure with time, as demonstrated by the absence of variation of pressure at

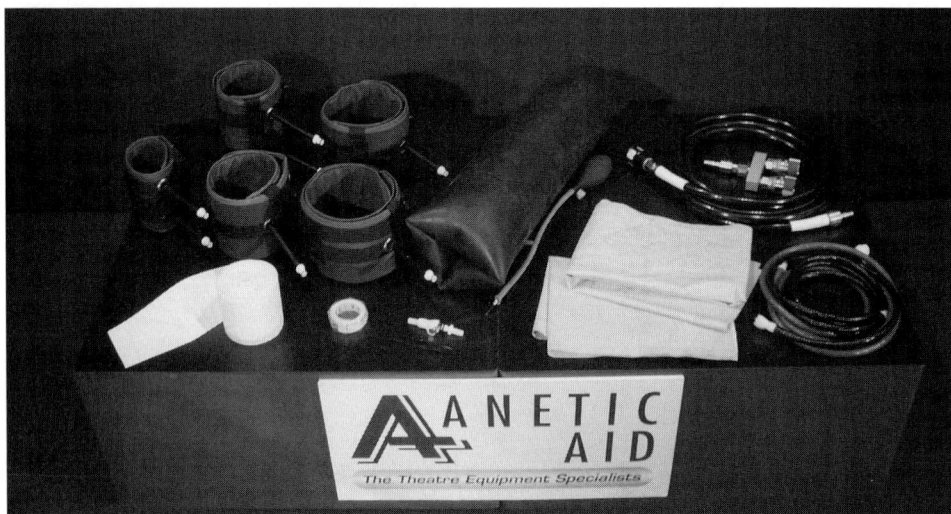

Figure 7.6 The variety of cuffs available with Rhys-Davies Exsanguinators. Reprinted courtesy of Anetic Aid, Guiseley, Leeds, UK.

400 mm Hg. Cuffs should exceed the circumference of the limb by 7–15 cm, should be of a width appropriate to the size of the patient (see Chapter 2), and should be positioned at the point of maximum circumference of the limb. As wide a cuff as possible should be selected.

Tourniquet time, site of application, and pressure must be recorded at the start of the operation, including the identification number of the specific tourniquet apparatus that was used. Once applied, the cuff should not be rotated into a new position, as this may cause a shearing injury. As described previously (see Chapters 2 and 5), fluid from skin preparations should not be allowed to collect under the cuff.

Additional care must be taken in bilateral procedures in which tourniquets are used on both limbs (see Chapter 2), since the risks of complications of the use of a tourniquet may be increased in such cases. The tourniquets should not be deflated simultaneously, but should be deflated separately with an interval of a few minutes to allow circulatory adjustment to the autotransfusion that occurs.

7.5 Practical Problems

The use of a bloodless field is integral to limb surgery, but it may have become a ritual. Stirling Bunnell stated[7]:

> It is impossible to dissect a hand properly without the aid of ischaemia from a tourniquet. It is also dangerous. Without a tourniquet the field is covered with blood, which is opaque; therefore instead of progressing with the dissection the surgeon will be

fumbling, traumatising the tissues by sponging constantly, and the tissues will be crushed by too many haemostats. Could a jeweller repair a watch immersed in ink? Dissection of a limb in which blood is held back by a tourniquet makes it possible to see every little nerve and vessel and to dissect with accuracy and minimal trauma.

At the other extreme, Jahss, the editor of a three-volume treatise on the foot and ankle, stated[8]: "We never use a tourniquet in adults, thereby avoiding tissue anoxia."

In contrast, Ward in 1976 reported a prospective, randomised trial in patients who required surgery for untreated Dupuytren's disease in the hand.[9] One group of patients were operated on using a tourniquet at 250 mm Hg after exsanguination of the limb. The hands of the other patients were treated on an elevated hand table without the use of a tourniquet. There were ten patients in each group, with an age range of 42–81 years. All patients had normotensive general anaesthesia. The same surgeon operated on all patients. It was found that when a tourniquet had been used, the hands remained significantly increased in volume compared with those operated upon without the use of a tourniquet. It was concluded that the use of the elevated hand table without a tourniquet placed no restrictions on the duration of surgery and also reduced the subsequent oedema. This technique was feasible but, as far as I am aware, has not been adopted elsewhere. It does illustrate, however, that a tourniquet is not mandatory, even for the hand.

Tzarnas has reported that carpal tunnel decompression can be performed safely under local anaesthesia.[10] The addition of a vasoconstrictor, adrenaline (epinephrine), to the local anaesthetic will cause sufficient vasoconstriction to maintain a dry field without the need for a tourniquet. A solution of 1% lidocaine and 1 : 100 000 adrenaline was injected into the line of the incision but not into the carpal tunnel to avoid injury to the median nerve. Initially, this technique was used for patients with arteriovenous fistulae for haemodialysis; later, its use was extended to other patients.

Similarly, there have been reports of randomised trials of tourniquet versus no tourniquet in 80 patients undergoing total knee replacement. Abdel-Salem and Eyres found a reduced complication rate after knee arthroplasty carried out without a tourniquet.[11] There was a significant reduction in postoperative pain, and knee movements were regained more rapidly. The authors did not have difficulty in creating a dry bone surface for the insertion of methylmethacrylate cement. In the tourniquet group, four patients had superficial wound sepsis and one had an area of skin necrosis that required grafting. Undertaking this operation without the use of a tourniquet may be useful in some patients with calcified vessels (see Chapter 5). However, a similar prospective, randomised trial in 77 patients found there was no significant difference in the surgical time, postoperative pain, need for analgesia, volume collected in the drains, postoperative swelling, or incidences of either wound complications or deep vein thrombosis.[12] The authors concluded that the use of a tourniquet is safe and current practice can be continued.

The use of a tourniquet for the internal fixation of fractures of the distal fibula has also been investigated.[13] Forty patients formed part of each group in a prospective, randomised trial. The operation time when using a tourniquet was significantly shorter (41±9 minutes) compared with not using a tourniquet (53±12 minutes). However, there were more complications when a tourniquet was used. Two patients in the tourniquet group had deep vein thrombosis of the calf. In the tourniquet group, seven patients had wound infections, compared with four in the no-tourniquet group. Patients in whom a tourniquet had not been used returned to work on average one week earlier than those in whom a tourniquet had been applied. The authors concluded that it is not justified to use a tourniquet in the operative treatment of simple, isolated fibular fractures.

Similarly, a randomised trial on 60 closed fractures of the tibia treated by open reduction and internal fixation with plates and screws was investigated.[14] Half the operations were performed with a thigh tourniquet and half were performed without. In the group in which tourniquets were used, there were six patients with erythema and induration of the wound; no such complications occurred in the no-tourniquet group. Despite negative cultures, superficial infection of the inflamed wounds was suspected. Surface swabs are known to be unreliable. It was suggested that the use of a tourniquet may predispose to infection, and their use was not recommended for internal fixation of the tibia.

The use of a tourniquet has also been questioned in arthroscopy of the knee. Two randomised trials have been reported, with opposite conclusions. In the first trial, 109 patients were investigated.[15] All patients had a tourniquet placed on the thigh and were assigned to have it either inflated or not inflated. There were two comparable groups. There was no significant difference between the two groups with respect to operative view, duration of operation, pain scores, analgesia requirements, or complications. The tourniquet required inflation during the operation in four patients who had been assigned to have it not inflated; in one patient, this made no difference to the operative view. It was concluded that the findings indicated that arthroscopy may be performed adequately without a tourniquet, and the authors recommended that the routine use of a tourniquet for this purpose be discontinued.

In the second trial, the authors reached the conclusion that the use of a pneumatic tourniquet at 300 mm Hg does not significantly affect the patient's quality of life or clinical outcome.[16] Visualisation was rated by surgeons to be three times better with a tourniquet than without, although operative time did not differ between the groups.

Another randomised trial of tourniquet use, mentioned in Chapter 5, reported on 48 patients undergoing anterior cruciate ligament reconstruction. This trial showed that use of a tourniquet for less than 114 minutes had no affect on the strength of the lower extremity after surgery.[17]

The questions surrounding exsanguination and use of tourniquets are controversial issues for arthroscopic surgery. A bloodless field provides an excellent view inside the knee. Surgical manipulations can be done without clouding of the image and troublesome bleeding. Nevertheless, as discussed above, a tourniquet is not necessary. A discriminatory approach is required, and this depends to a large extent on the surgeon's preference. Not using a tourniquet may save time, produces no reactive hyperaemia, and carries less risk of postoperative bleeding. It may be necessary to selectively coagulate bleeding sites. Minor bleeding from the skin incision for the arthroscopic portal is prevented by infiltration with local anaesthetic and adrenaline.

7.5.1 Use of Tourniquets in Cases of Trauma

The tourniquet plays a limited but important role in the management of open fractures and severe hand injuries.[18] Proper use of a tourniquet in debridement of open fractures is essential. An open fracture is usually a high-energy injury; the debridement, apart from cleansing, involves removing dead and devitalised tissue from living tissue. It is argued that intramedullary bleeding is not obscured by an inflated tourniquet, but this misses the point: what is of value is the vascularity of soft-tissue pedicles to butterfly fragments. Without a tourniquet, it is easy to identify such pedicles when they are clearly non-viable and as such declare the attached butterfly as dead. In the presence of a tourniquet, one invariably declares such a butterfly fragment as viable purely on the strength of a pedicle being present, irrespective of any blood flow within it. Perhaps it may be a comprise to suggest that a tourniquet may be applied but not inflated unless unexpected bleeding is encountered, when it is necessary to control bleeding to allow a clear view or to limit blood loss. The anoxia that is produced by a tourniquet also interferes with the assessment of the viability of muscle and may add to a pre-existing ischaemic injury. Nevertheless, inflation for ten minutes followed by release produces a capillary flush of the skin distal to the tourniquet, which is a helpful indicator of skin viability. This also allows the identification of neurovascular structures, particularly in the upper limb. A tourniquet is not required for intramedullary nailing, since it may potentiate thermal necrosis of bone.

It has also been shown that in multiply injured patients, the combination of reamed femoral nailing with fracture fixation under tourniquet control increases pulmonary morbidity.[19] The data from a retrospective review show that multiply injured patients have an increased length of dependence on a ventilator and a longer stay in the intensive care unit. It is suggested that tourniquets should not be used routinely in this situation and, if necessary, total tourniquet time should be minimised.

Many surgeons routinely use pneumatic tourniquets in ankle fractures. A bloodless field facilitates anatomical reduction and may reduce the time for surgery. The use of a tourniquet in such cases may result in more postoperative pain and a higher incidence of wound infections. Using a slight Trendelenburg position of the operation table will reduce bleeding and avoid the need for a tourniquet.

7.5.2 Drug Kinetics

A tourniquet can reduce the penetration of antibiotics into distal tissues, and the optimal time interval between administration of a prophylactic antibiotic and inflation of the tourniquet is important. Intravenous administration in the operating theatre ensures peak tissue levels at the time of surgery. Bannister and colleagues measured antibiotic levels in bone and fat in patients having knee replacements to determine the time that should elapse between the intravenous injection of the antibiotic and inflation of the tourniquet.[20] The tissue levels increased progressively with time, and there was wide variation in absorption rate between patients and between the two cephalosporins assessed. Five minutes is a safe time between systemic injection and inflation of the tourniquet. It was recommended that the antibiotic be given intravenously at an early stage of induction of anaesthesia.

7.5.3 Application of the Cuff

When the cuff is applied to the limb, it is usual to cover the site with a layer of plaster wool, applied carefully with no folds, i.e. wrinkle-free. An alternative has been described, in which a piece of stockinet wrapping, three times the width of the tourniquet, is placed on the limb.[21] The tourniquet is applied firmly and the fastenings are secured. The stockinet is then folded and a small cut is made to allow passage of the air connection. Due to the elasticity of the stockinet, the tourniquet is held in place when inflated. There may be some difficulty in achieving a secure proximal position in obese patients. The patients who present the greatest difficulty are those who have copious subcutaneous, loose, flabby fat. Obese patients frequently require a relatively longer incision for adequate exposure at operation, so a more proximal position is important. The manoeuvre described by Krackow is achieved simply by having an assistant grasp the flesh just below the site where the tourniquet is to be applied and firmly pulling this loose tissue distally before the plaster wool is applied.[22] Traction on the soft tissue is maintained while the tourniquet is applied and secured. When the flesh is released, the bulky tissue supports the tourniquet and pushes it into a more proximal position. Excessive tightening of the tourniquet must be avoided, since it does not help to maintain the proximal position of the tourniquet but creates the effect of a venous tourniquet, which increases bleeding when the tourniquet is deflated at the end of an operation. Using this technique, the tourniquet may be positioned securely 10–15 cm more proximally on the fat thigh. A similar technique can be used on the upper limb.

7.5.4 Release of the Tourniquet and Wound Closure

Opinion is divided as to the timing of removal of a tourniquet. Some surgeons maintain the inflation of the tourniquet while closing the wound and applying a pressure dressing, releasing the tourniquet as the final step in the operation. Others release the tourniquet before wound closure to identify bleeding points and control haemorrhage before closing the wound and applying a pressure dressing. The latter believe that their more elaborate approach minimises the risk of postoperative haematoma and the oedema. Himel and colleagues tested the effects of the two techniques in a series of rabbits having standardised operations on both lower limbs.[23] The animals were injected with 99m technetium-labelled red cells and scanned to measure haematoma formation. It was concluded that the release of a tourniquet after wound closure was associated with greater haematoma formation. A similar conclusion was reached by Mars in an experimental investigation in a primate model.[24] The common practice of closing a wound and applying a compression bandage before deflation of the tourniquet was shown to raise intracompartmental pressure. When the tourniquet was released, a further rise occurred. Postoperative intracompartmental pressure remained significantly higher during the first three hours of reperfusion in limbs bandaged before release of the tourniquet, rather than in those in which the tourniquet was released and haemostasis secured before the limb was bandaged.[25]

The effect of timing the release of the tourniquet on blood loss was investigated in 81 patients undergoing knee replacements.[26] The patients were allocated randomly to one of two groups. In one group, the tourniquet was released for haemostasis before wound closure; in the other group, the tourniquet was not released until the wound was closed and a pressure dressing had been applied. No difference was found in total blood loss between the two groups. Nevertheless, with a large wound, early release of the tourniquet does give the opportunity to ensure that there is no major bleeding before the wound is sutured.

7.6 Golden Rules for the Safe Use of Tourniquets

To paraphrase Voltaire, "the price of safety is eternal vigilance". Tourniquet time is precious and must be used economically.

1   Only use a tourniquet on a limb with a normal, blood supply.

2   Always use a pneumatic tourniquet. Be sure that the gauge has been checked and is correct.

3   Beware of thin, atrophied limbs. Apply protective padding without wrinkles.

4   Three hours is the final upper limit of safety, but try to keep well within this time. The pressure applied to the limb is just as important as the duration of ischaemia: it should be related to the patient's blood pressure, the lowest effective pressure being used.

5   Do not exsanguinate the limb by external compression in the presence of suspected malignancy or infection.

6   Bilateral tourniquets can be a hazard in patients with poor left ventricular function.

7   There is no benefit from using breathing periods. Keep the tourniquet inflated for as long as required, but do not exceed three hours. Once the tourniquet has been released, it should not be reinflated.

8   Remember that limbs always swell after a tourniquet has been used. Reduce swelling to a minimum by releasing the tourniquet before suture of the wound where practicable. Never apply a complete plaster after the use of a tourniquet.

9   Release the tourniquet routinely before closing large wounds in order to secure haemostasis.

10 Check carefully that the circulation has returned to all digits after the plaster or bandage has been applied.

11 Seal off the tourniquet from the wound to prevent soaking of padding.

12 Always record the times of application and release of the tourniquet, the pressure, and the number of the tourniquet used.

References

1   Department of Health and Social Security (1985). Evaluation of pneumatic tourniquet controllers. Health Equipment Information Number 138. London: Department of Health and Social Security.

2   Durkin, MAP, Crabtree, SD (1982). Hazard of pneumatic tourniquet application. *Proceedings of the Royal Society of Medicine* **75**: 658–660.

3   Association of Operating Room Nurses (1990). Recommended practices. *American Operating Room Nurses Journal* **52**: 1041–1043.

4   Prevoznik, SJ (1970). Injury from use of pneumatic tourniquet. *Journal of Anaesthesiology* **32**: 177.

5   Klenerman, L (1983). Tourniquet paralysis. *Journal of Bone and Joint Surgery* **65B**: 374–375.

6   Hallett, J (1983). Inaccurate tourniquet gauges. *British Medical Journal* **286**: 1267.

7   Boyes, JH, ed. (1964). *Bunnell's Surgery of the Hand*, 4th edn. London: Pitman Medial, p. 132.

8   Jahss, MH, ed. (1991). *Disorders of the Foot and Ankle*, 2nd edn. Philadelphia: W.B. Saunders Co.

9   Ward, GM (1976). Oedema of the hand after fasciectomy with or without tourniquet. *Hand* **8**: 179–185.

10 Tzarnas, CD (1993). Carpal tunnel release without a tourniquet. *Journal of Hand Surgery* **18A**: 1041–1043.

11 Abdel-Salam, A, Eyres, KS (1995). Effects of tourniquet during total knee arthroplasty. *Journal of Bone and Joint Surgery* **77B**: 250–253.

12 Wakanker, HM, Nicholl, JE, Koka, R, D'Arcy, JC (1999). The tourniquet in knee arthroplasty. *Journal of Bone and Joint Surgery* **81B**: 30–33.

13 Maffulli, N, Testa, V, Capesso, G (1993). Use of a tourniquet in the internal fixation of the distal part of the fibula. *Journal of Bone and Joint Surgery* **75A**: 700–703.

14 Salam, AA, Eyres, KS, Cleary, J, El-Sayed, HH (1991). The use of a tourniquet when plating tibial fractures. *Journal of Bone and Joint Surgery* **73B**: 86–87.

15 Johnson, DS, Stewart, H, Hirst, P, Harper, NJN (2000). Is tourniquet use necessary for arthroscopy? *Journal of Arthroscopic and Related Surgery* **16**: 648–651.

16 Kirkley, A, Rampersaud, R, Griffin, S, et al. (2000). Tourniquet versus no tourniquet use in routine knee arthroscopy: a prospective, double-blind, randomised clinical trial. *Journal of Arthroscopic and Related Surgery* **16**: 121–126.

17 Nicholas, SJ, Tyler, TF, McHugh, MP, Gleim, GW (2001). Effects on leg strength of tourniquet use during anterior cruciate ligament reconstruction. A prospective randomised study. *Journal of Arthroscopic and Related Surgery* **17**: 603–607.

18 Bucholz, RW, Heckman, J, eds. (2001). *Rockwood and Green's Fractures in Adults*. Philadelphia: Lippincott, Williams & Wilkins, p. 294.

19 Pollak, AN, Battistella, F, Pelteg, J, et al. (1997). Reamed femoral nailing in patients with multiple injuries. Adverse affects of tourniquet use. *Clinical Orthopaedics and Related Research* **339**: 41–46.

20 Bannister, GC, Auchencloss, JM, Johnson, DP, Newman, JH (1988). The timing of tourniquet application in relation to prophylactic antibiotic administration. *Journal of Bone and Joint Surgery* **70B**: 322–324.

21 Harland, P, Lovell, ME (1994). An alternative method of tourniquet padding. *Annals of the Royal College of Surgeons* **76**: 107.

22 Krackow, KA (1982). A manoeuvre for improved positioning of tourniquet in the obese patient. *Clinical Orthopaedics and Related Research* **168**: 80–82.

23 Himel, HN, Ahmed, M, Parmett, SR, et al. (1989). Effect of the timing of tourniquet release on postoperative haematoma formation: an experimental animal study. *Plastic and Reconstructive Surgery* **83**: 692–697.

24 Mars, M (1994). The effect of postoperative bleeding on compartment pressure. *Journal of Hand Surgery* **19B**: 149–153.

25 Mars, M, Brock-Utne, JG (1991). The effect of tourniquet release on intra-compartmental pressure in the bandaged and unbandaged limb. *Journal of Hand Surgery* **16B**, 318–322.

26 Widman, J, Isacson, J (1999). Surgical haemostasis after tourniquet release does not reduce blood loss in knee replacement. *Acta Orthopaedica Scandinavica* **70**: 268–270.

Index